NATIONAL ACADEMIES Sciences Engineering Medicine

NATIONAL ACADEMIES PRESS
Washington, DC

Developing a Multidisciplinary and Multispecialty Workforce for Patients with Cancer, from Diagnosis to Survivorship

Erin Balogh, Laurene Graig, Anne Johnson, and Sharyl Nass,
Rapporteurs

National Cancer Policy Forum

Board on Health Care Services

Global Forum on Innovation in Health Professional Education

Board on Global Health

Health and Medicine Division

Proceedings of a Workshop

NATIONAL ACADEMIES PRESS 500 Fifth Street, NW Washington, DC 20001

This activity was supported by Contract No. 75D30121D11240 (Task Order Nos. 75D30121F00002 and 75D30123F00024) and Contract No. HHSN263201800029I (Task Order Nos. HHSN26300008 and 75N98023F00019) with the Centers for Disease Control and Prevention and the National Cancer Institute/National Institutes of Health, respectively, and by the American Association for Cancer Research; American Cancer Society; American College of Radiology; American Society of Clinical Oncology; Association of American Cancer Institutes; Association of Community Cancer Centers; Flatiron Health; Merck & Co., Inc.; National Comprehensive Cancer Network; National Patient Advocate Foundation; Novartis Oncology; Oncology Nursing Society; Partners in Health; Pfizer Inc.; Sanofi; and Society for Immunotherapy of Cancer. Any opinions, findings, conclusions, or recommendations expressed in this publication do not necessarily reflect the views of any organization or agency that provided support for the project.

International Standard Book Number-13: 978-0-309-71912-4
International Standard Book Number-10: 0-309-71912-7
Digital Object Identifier: https://doi.org/10.17226/27769

This publication is available from the National Academies Press, 500 Fifth Street, NW, Keck 360, Washington, DC 20001; (800) 624-6242 or (202) 334-3313; http://www.nap.edu.

Copyright 2024 by the National Academy of Sciences. National Academies of Sciences, Engineering, and Medicine and National Academies Press and the graphical logos for each are all trademarks of the National Academies of Sciences. All rights reserved.

Printed in the United States of America.

Suggested citation: National Academies of Sciences, Engineering, and Medicine. 2024. *Developing a multidisciplinary and multispecialty workforce for patients with cancer, from diagnosis to survivorship: Proceedings of a workshop.* Washington, DC: The National Academies Press. https://doi.org/10.17226/27769.

The **National Academy of Sciences** was established in 1863 by an Act of Congress, signed by President Lincoln, as a private, nongovernmental institution to advise the nation on issues related to science and technology. Members are elected by their peers for outstanding contributions to research. Dr. Marcia McNutt is president.

The **National Academy of Engineering** was established in 1964 under the charter of the National Academy of Sciences to bring the practices of engineering to advising the nation. Members are elected by their peers for extraordinary contributions to engineering. Dr. John L. Anderson is president.

The **National Academy of Medicine** (formerly the Institute of Medicine) was established in 1970 under the charter of the National Academy of Sciences to advise the nation on medical and health issues. Members are elected by their peers for distinguished contributions to medicine and health. Dr. Victor J. Dzau is president.

The three Academies work together as the **National Academies of Sciences, Engineering, and Medicine** to provide independent, objective analysis and advice to the nation and conduct other activities to solve complex problems and inform public policy decisions. The National Academies also encourage education and research, recognize outstanding contributions to knowledge, and increase public understanding in matters of science, engineering, and medicine.

Learn more about the National Academies of Sciences, Engineering, and Medicine at **www.nationalacademies.org**.

Consensus Study Reports published by the National Academies of Sciences, Engineering, and Medicine document the evidence-based consensus on the study's statement of task by an authoring committee of experts. Reports typically include findings, conclusions, and recommendations based on information gathered by the committee and the committee's deliberations. Each report has been subjected to a rigorous and independent peer-review process and it represents the position of the National Academies on the statement of task.

Proceedings published by the National Academies of Sciences, Engineering, and Medicine chronicle the presentations and discussions at a workshop, symposium, or other event convened by the National Academies. The statements and opinions contained in proceedings are those of the participants and are not endorsed by other participants, the planning committee, or the National Academies.

Rapid Expert Consultations published by the National Academies of Sciences, Engineering, and Medicine are authored by subject-matter experts on narrowly focused topics that can be supported by a body of evidence. The discussions contained in rapid expert consultations are considered those of the authors and do not contain policy recommendations. Rapid expert consultations are reviewed by the institution before release.

For information about other products and activities of the National Academies, please visit www.nationalacademies.org/about/whatwedo.

PLANNING COMMITTEE[1]

LARISSA NEKHLYUDOV (*Co-Chair*), Brigham and Women's Hospital; Dana-Farber Cancer Institute; Harvard Medical School
LAWRENCE N. SHULMAN (*Co-Chair*), University of Pennsylvania
KAREN BASEN-ENGQUIST, The University of Texas MD Anderson Cancer Center
SMITA BHATIA, University of Alabama, Birmingham
ROBERT CARLSON, National Comprehensive Cancer Network
GWEN DARIEN, National Patient Advocate Foundation
ANITA GUPTA, Johns Hopkins University
CHANITA HUGHES-HALBERT, University of Southern California
RANDY A. JONES, University of Virginia
RANDALL A. OYER, University of Pennsylvania; Penn Medicine Lancaster General Health
SUSAN M. SCHNEIDER, Duke University
ROBERT A. WINN, Virginia Commonwealth University
ROBIN YABROFF, American Cancer Society

Project Staff

ANNA ADLER, Senior Program Assistant (*from September 2023*)
LORI BENJAMIN BRENIG, Research Associate (*until May 2023*)
TORRIE BROWN, Program Coordinator
CHIDINMA CHUKWURAH, Senior Program Assistant (*until April 2024*)
EMMA WICKLAND, Research Associate (*from September 2023*)
JULIE WILTSHIRE, Senior Finance Business Partner
JENNIFER ZHU, Associate Program Officer
PATRICIA CUFF, Director, Global Forum on Innovation in Health Professional Education
ERIN BALOGH, Co-Director, National Cancer Policy Forum (*until June 2024*)
LAURENE GRAIG, Senior Program Officer (*June–July 2024*)

---

[1] The National Academies of Sciences, Engineering, and Medicine's planning committees are solely responsible for organizing the workshop, identifying topics, and choosing speakers. The responsibility for the published Proceedings of a Workshop rests with the workshop rapporteurs and the institution.

FRANCIS AMANKWAH, Co-Director, National Cancer Policy Forum (*from July 2024*)
SHARYL NASS, Co-Director, National Cancer Policy Forum; Senior Director, Board on Health Care Services

NATIONAL CANCER POLICY FORUM[1]

ROBERT A. WINN (*Chair*), Virginia Commonwealth University
PETER C. ADAMSON, Sanofi
JUSTIN E. BEKELMAN, University of Pennsylvania
SMITA BHATIA, The University of Alabama at Birmingham
GIDEON BLUMENTHAL, Merck
CHRIS BOSHOFF, Pfizer Inc.
OTIS W. BRAWLEY, Johns Hopkins University
CHRISTINA CHAPMAN, Baylor College of Medicine; Michael E. DeBakey VA Medical Center
GWEN DARIEN, National Patient Advocate Foundation
CRYSTAL DENLINGER, National Comprehensive Cancer Network
JAMES H. DOROSHOW, National Cancer Institute
S. GAIL ECKHARDT, The University of Texas at Austin
CHRISTOPHER R. FRIESE, University of Michigan
STANTON L. GERSON, Case Western Reserve University
SCARLETT LIN GOMEZ, University of California, San Francisco
JULIE R. GRALOW, American Society of Clinical Oncology
ROY S. HERBST, Yale University; American Association for Cancer Research
HEDVIG HRICAK, Memorial Sloan Kettering Cancer Center
CHANITA HUGHES-HALBERT, University of Southern California
ROY A. JENSEN, University of Kansas; Association of American Cancer Institutes
RANDY A. JONES, University of Virginia
BETH Y. KARLAN, University of California, Los Angeles
SAMIR N. KHLEIF, Georgetown University; Society for Immunotherapy of Cancer
SCOTT M. LIPPMAN, University of California, San Diego
ELENA MARTINEZ, University of California, San Diego
LARISSA NEKHLYUDOV, Brigham and Women's Hospital; Dana-Farber Cancer Institute; Harvard Medical School

---

[1] The National Academies of Sciences, Engineering, and Medicine's forums and roundtables do not issue, review, or approve individual documents. The responsibility for the published Proceedings of a Workshop rests with the workshop rapporteurs and the institution.

RANDALL A. OYER, University of Pennsylvania; Penn Medicine Lancaster General Health; Association of Community Cancer Centers
CLEO A. RYALS, Flatiron Health
RICHARD L. SCHILSKY, ASCO TAPUR Study; University of Chicago
JULIE SCHNEIDER, Oncology Center of Excellence, U.S. Food and Drug Administration
SUSAN M. SCHNEIDER, Duke University
LAWRENCE N. SHULMAN, University of Pennsylvania
HEIDI SMITH, Novartis Pharmaceuticals
KATRINA TRIVERS, Centers for Disease Control and Prevention
ROBIN YABROFF, American Cancer Society

Forum Staff

ANNA ADLER, Senior Program Assistant
TORRIE BROWN, Program Coordinator
CHIDINMA CHUKWURAH, Senior Program Assistant (*until April 2024*)
EMMA WICKLAND, Research Associate
JULIE WILTSHIRE, Senior Finance Business Partner
JENNIFER ZHU, Associate Program Officer
ERIN BALOGH, Co-Director, National Cancer Policy Forum (*until June 2024*)
LAURENE GRAIG, Senior Program Officer (*June–July 2024*)
FRANCIS AMANKWAH, Co-Director, National Cancer Policy Forum (*from July 2024*)
SHARYL NASS, Co-Director, National Cancer Policy Forum; Senior Director, Board on Health Care Services

Reviewers

This Proceedings of a Workshop was reviewed in draft form by individuals chosen for their diverse perspectives and technical expertise. The purpose of this independent review is to provide candid and critical comments that will assist the National Academies of Sciences, Engineering, and Medicine in making each published proceedings as sound as possible and to ensure that it meets the institutional standards for quality, objectivity, evidence, and responsiveness to the charge. The review comments and draft manuscript remain confidential to protect the integrity of the process.

We thank the following individuals for their review of this report:

DAVID DOUGHERTY, University of Pennsylvania
HILARY Y. MA, MD Anderson Cancer Center
WILLIAM PIRL, Harvard Medical School

Although the reviewers listed above provided many constructive comments and suggestions, they were not asked to endorse the conclusions or recommendations of this report nor did they see the final draft before its release. The review of this proceedings was overseen by **PATRICIA GANZ,** University of California, Los Angeles. She was responsible for making certain that an independent examination of this report was carried out in accordance with the standards of the National Academies and that all review comments were carefully considered. Responsibility for the final content rests entirely with the rapporteurs and the National Academies.

We also thank staff member Abigail Allen for reading and providing helpful comments on this manuscript.

Acknowledgments

The National Cancer Policy Forum is grateful for the support of our many annual sponsors. Federal sponsors include the Centers for Disease Control and Prevention and the National Cancer Institute/National Institutes of Health. Nonfederal sponsors include the American Association for Cancer Research; American Cancer Society; American College of Radiology; American Society of Clinical Oncology; Association of American Cancer Institutes; Association of Community Cancer Centers; Flatiron Health; Merck & Co., Inc.; National Comprehensive Cancer Network; National Patient Advocate Foundation; Novartis Oncology; Oncology Nursing Society; Partners in Health; Pfizer Inc.; Sanofi; and Society for Immunotherapy of Cancer.

The forum wishes to express its gratitude to the expert speakers whose presentations and discussions helped inform efforts to improve equitable access to multispeciality, multidisciplinary care for patients living with and beyond cancer. The forum also wishes to thank the members of the planning committee for their work in developing an excellent workshop agenda.

Contents

Acronyms and Abbreviations	xvii
Proceedings of a Workshop	1
WORKSHOP OVERVIEW	1
IMPROVING MULTIDISCIPLINARY AND MULTISPECIALTY CARE IN THE CANCER CARE CONTINUUM	3

    Common Challenges Facing Cancer Survivors, 3
    The Role of Specialty Care and the Need for Coordination, 11
    Addressing Disparities, 22
    Advancing Multidisciplinary, Multispecialty Care, 23

EDUCATION AND TRAINING OPPORTUNITIES	25

    Interprofessional Collaborative Practice and Interprofessional Education, 25
    The Cancer and Aging Research Group: An Education and Training Network to Facilitate Multidisciplinary, Multispecialty Expert Care, 27
    Project ECHO: Capacity Building for PCPs in Cancer Survivorship Care, 29
    ENGAGE: Person-Centered Coordinated Care at the Intersection of Cancer and Mental Health, 30
    Supporting Training to Prioritize Access to Care, 31

HEALTH SYSTEM OPPORTUNITIES 31
    The Impetus and Challenge of System-Level Interventions to Support Survivorship, 32
    Integration of Health Systems for Better Cancer Survivorship Care, 34
    Leveraging Data and Technology, 35
    Learning from Other Fields of Medicine, 36
    System-Level Efforts to Reduce Health Disparities, 37

POLICY, PAYMENT, AND ADVOCACY OPPORTUNITIES 38
    The Human Toll of Policy and Payment Challenges, 38
    Closing Gaps in Insurance Coverage for Survivorship Care, 39
    Ideas and Efforts to Improve Payment and Service Delivery Models, 42
    Policy Options to Facilitate Care Coordination and Navigation, 43
    Alternative Payment Models, 44
    The Power of Perceptions of Value on Patient-, Clinician-, and System-Level Decisions, 45
    Facilitating Effective Team-Based Care, 45
    The Quest for Equity, 46

CLOSING DISCUSSION 46
REFERENCES 48

APPENDIXES
A   Statement of Task 61
B   Workshop Agenda 63

Boxes and Figures

BOXES

1 Observations from Individual Workshop Speakers Regarding the Importance and Challenges of Providing Multidisciplinary, Multispecialty Care for Cancer Survivors, 4
2 Suggestions from Individual Workshop Speakers Regarding Ways to Improve the Provision of Multidisciplinary, Multispecialty Care for Cancer Survivors, 5
3 Experiences Shared by Cancer Survivors, 8

FIGURES

1 U.S. cancer survivors by years from diagnosis, 10
2 Strategies to mitigate inequities and disparities at the intersection of cardiovascular disease and cancer, 14
3 An example risk stratification workflow for cancer survivorship care, 19
4 Conceptual schematic illustrating an example of a multiteam framework for collaborative cancer care, 28
5 Conceptual diagram highlighting areas for which return on investment (ROI) from efforts to improve survivorship care can be assessed across the health system, 33
6 Five-year survival following cancer diagnosis in the United States by socioeconomic status quintile, 39
7 Percentage of adults age 19–64 years without health insurance coverage by state in 2019, 40

Acronyms and Abbreviations

ACA	Affordable Care Act
AI	artificial intelligence
APP	advanced practice provider
ASCO	American Society of Clinical Oncology
CARG	Cancer and Aging Research Group
CHC	community health center
CHOP	Children's Hospital of Pennsylvania
CMS	Centers for Medicare & Medicaid Services
CoC	Commission on Cancer
CVD	cardiovascular disease
ECANA	Endometrial Cancer Action Network for African Americans
ECHO	Extension of Community Health Outcomes
EHR	electronic health record
EOM	Enhancing Oncology Model
ePRO	electronic patient-reported outcome
FQHC	federally qualified health center
IPCP	interprofessional collaborative practice
IPE	interprofessional education
ML	machine learning

NCCN	National Comprehensive Cancer Network
NCI	National Cancer Institute
NLP	natural language processing
PCP	primary care provider/physician
PRO	patient-reported outcome
PT	physical therapy/therapist
SDOH	social determinants of health

Proceedings of a Workshop

WORKSHOP OVERVIEW[1]

People living with and beyond cancer require multidisciplinary, multi-specialty care to address a broad range of health care needs—from monitoring for cancer recurrence to detecting and managing toxicities to addressing psychosocial challenges—that affect their health and well-being throughout their lives. However, many people face significant barriers in accessing the specialized medical expertise they need, navigating systems of referrals and payments, and receiving care that is appropriately comprehensive and coordinated, said Larissa Nekhlyudov, clinical director of internal medicine for cancer survivors at Brigham and Women's Hospital/Dana-Farber Cancer Institute and professor of medicine at Harvard Medical School. She added that many of the clinicians and institutions caring for people with cancer and cancer survivors face substantial challenges in identifying and addressing complex care needs, keeping pace with the high level of demand for care given workforce shortages and gaps in access to specialized expertise, and forming and sustaining effective care teams across specialties and clinical practices.

---

[1] This workshop was organized by an independent planning committee whose role was limited to identification of topics and speakers. This Proceedings of a Workshop was prepared by the rapporteurs as a factual summary of the presentations and discussions that took place at the workshop. Statements, recommendations, and opinions expressed are those of individual presenters and participants and are not endorsed or verified by the National Academies of Sciences, Engineering, and Medicine, and they should not be construed as reflecting any group consensus.

To examine opportunities to improve equitable access to multidisciplinary, multispecialty care for cancer survivors, the National Cancer Policy Forum and the Global Forum on Innovation in Health Professional Education of the National Academies of Sciences, Engineering, and Medicine hosted a workshop, Developing a Multidisciplinary and Multispecialty Workforce for Patients with Cancer, from Diagnosis to Survivorship. It was held on July 17–18, 2023, and convened experts in clinical care, cancer research, health care policy, patient advocacy, and related areas.

More people are living with and beyond cancer, due in part to an increase in cancer diagnoses and better survival rates brought about by medical advancements and innovative therapies, said Lawrence Shulman, director of the Center for Global Cancer Medicine at the University of Pennsylvania Abramson Cancer Center, who outlined the goals of the workshop. He explained that many people with a history of cancer are now living decades past their initial diagnosis, are in older age groups, and have one or more comorbidities, often related to the effects of their cancer treatment. To navigate through diagnosis, treatment, and long-term survivorship, people need informed, attentive, and coordinated health care from a wide range of health care professionals (Bluethmann et al., 2016). However, this multidisciplinary, multispecialty collaborative care is highly complex and remains difficult to obtain and coordinate, Shulman said.

Much of the focus and energy in cancer research centers around emerging treatments, but it is vital to recognize that every new treatment may be associated with its own set of side effects—some of which may not be evident for decades, said Robert Winn, the director of the VCU Massey Comprehensive Cancer Center at Virginia Commonwealth University. Whatever promise new treatments may hold, it is essential for the health care system to do a better job of meeting the needs of survivors, he emphasized, cautioning that "innovation does not always equal impact." Winn underscored the importance of remaining grounded in the core value of doing good, which requires recognizing and mitigating potential harms.

Although cancer treatments are intended to extend life and improve quality of life, it is important to recognize that they also can cause harm. Posttreatment complications can occur with any cancer treatment and last for decades, affect survival rates, and increase the likelihood of a second cancer, Shulman noted (Meyer et al., 2012; Schaapveld et al., 2015). Indeed, many cancer survivors report profound functional limitations decades after treatment, particularly older adults. In addition, while short-term organ toxicity of cancer therapies is often well characterized, many newer treatments do not have a long history of use, so data are profoundly lacking on long-term effects needed to inform treatment decisions and survivorship care. Shulman explained that some toxicities can take years to appear or may increase over time, so the typical 5 years of follow-up care is inadequate to identify, understand, and address these potential issues (Patel et al., 2023).

Many speakers examined the challenges that patients, their caregivers, and health systems face in achieving proactive, comprehensive, and coordinated survivorship care (see Box 1). Many speakers also described opportunities to create pathways and systems to provide better, more collaborative, and more holistic care for patients with cancer, from diagnosis onward (see Box 2). Appendixes A and B include the workshop Statement of Task and agenda, respectively. Speaker presentations and the workshop recordings have been archived online.[2]

IMPROVING MULTIDISCIPLINARY AND MULTISPECIALTY CARE IN THE CANCER CARE CONTINUUM

The workshop examined the challenges that cancer survivors face in managing health issues related to their cancer and cancer treatment and how multidisciplinary, multispecialty care can address these issues across the lifespan. Drawing upon research findings, patient experiences, and perspectives from specialists in a variety of areas, speakers discussed key gaps, opportunities, and considerations to lay the groundwork for improving the provision and coordination of survivorship care

Common Challenges Facing Cancer Survivors

Shulman defined a cancer survivor[3] as any person with a history of cancer, from the time of diagnosis through the remainder of their life. This can include people who live with cancer continuously, people with intermittent periods of active disease, and people free of cancer. Many cancer survivors experience complications from treatment, often years or decades later, and some also experience a cancer recurrence or second cancer. This complexity and variation was highlighted by several people who shared their lived experiences of cancer treatment and survivorship care (see Box 3).

The population of cancer survivors is large, growing, and aging. It is projected that the United States will have more than 22 million cancer survivors by 2030, noted Robert Carlson, chief executive officer at the National Comprehensive Cancer Network (NCCN), and Linda Jacobs, clinical professor

---

[2] See https://www.nationalacademies.org/event/07-17-2023/developing-a-multidisciplinary-and-multispecialty-workforce-for-patients-with-cancer-from-diagnosis-to-survivorship-a-workshop (accessed January 8, 2024).

[3] See https://cancercontrol.cancer.gov/ocs/definitions (accessed March 27, 2024).

BOX 1
Observations from Individual Workshop Speakers Regarding the Importance and Challenges of Providing Multidisciplinary, Multispecialty Care for Cancer Survivors

Overburdened and underdeveloped health systems
- The population of cancer survivors is large, growing, and aging. Many people with a history of cancer are now living decades past their initial diagnosis and have one or more comorbidities, often related to the effects of their cancer treatment. (Carlson, Jacobs, Klepin, Shulman)
- The number of cancer survivors in need of specialty care is growing more rapidly than the number of specialists. (Carlson, Jacobs, Mayer, Shulman)
- Health issues related to cancer treatment are often overlooked until they become crises due to lack of screening and referrals. (Irwin, Meacham, Pirl, Thomson, Von Ah)

Disparities and inequitable access to care
- Social determinants of health, costs of care and insurance limitations, and systemic issues with health care access contribute to disparities in cancer and survivorship care outcomes. (Irwin, Pirl, Winn, Yabroff)
- Although new cancer treatments often attract the most attention, it is equally if not more important to ensure the effective and equitable delivery of existing treatments and survivorship care. (Kamal, Winn)
- Patients need adequate information about the potential benefits and risks of cancer treatments to make informed decisions that align with their treatment and life goals. (Dusetzina, Gracia, Perkins, Winn)

Challenges with interdisciplinary care collaboration for cancer survivors
- Even medical centers that have access to specialists face challenges in integrating them into an effective, collaborative care team focused on survivorship. (Jacobs, Mayer)
- Certain financial models, such as fee-for-service reimbursement, do not support complex care coordination, and most health systems lack structures to support team-based care across disciplines and locations or with external organizations. (Dougherty)

> **BOX 1 Continued**
>
> NOTE: This list is the rapporteurs' synopsis of observations made by one or more individual speakers as identified. These statements have not been endorsed or verified by the National Academies of Sciences, Engineering, and Medicine. They are not intended to reflect a consensus among workshop participants.

> **BOX 2**
> **Suggestions from Individual Workshop Speakers Regarding Ways to Improve the Provision of Multidisciplinary, Multispecialty Care for Cancer Survivors**
>
> **Enhancing patient outcomes through innovative technology and interventions**
> - Use risk stratification to guide coordinated, multispecialty interventions and integrate specialist care into treatment and follow-up decisions. (Alfano, Choi, Ky)
> - Use electronic health records (EHRs) and other tools to prioritize, incentivize, and leverage structured, standardized, interoperable, and shareable data to improve multidisciplinary, risk-stratified, evidence-based clinical care navigation. (Alfano, Brasfield, Dougherty, Shulman, Tevaarwerk)
> - Advance innovative, embedded, collaborative, and consultative care models in which specialists do not have to compete for resources to optimize patient care. (Reid)
> - Harness new technologies, such as machine learning and artificial intelligence, to "work smarter" and streamline patient–clinician interactions, screen for unmet needs, and tailor care to each individual situation, while working to ensure that these technologies do not perpetuate bias or exacerbate disparities. (Darien, Mayer, Tevaarwerk, Winn)
>
> *continued*

BOX 2 Continued

Enhancing clinician education
- Develop and fund educational and training programs that focus on interprofessional, team-based care and competencies to support cancer survivorship. (Brasfield, Choi, Gracia, Gupta, Heflin, Jacobs, Klepin, Mayer, Weaver)
- Replace board exams with more frequent and structured learning modules that can better incorporate emerging research and best practices. (Brasfield)
- Engage, elevate, and activate community health centers through culturally tailored and effective education, training, and navigation to develop survivorship roadmaps and community-based referral pathways. (Allicock, Reid, Winn)

Developing multidisciplinary clinical teams
- Use a stepped-care approach to support the efficient use of resources in screening, tracking, and incorporating mental health care with medical care. (Pirl)
- Integrate nutrition into patient-centered care, including screening tools embedded in EHRs, telehealth, insurance coverage, patient communication, and research funding. (Thomson)
- Include primary care clinician in patients' multidisciplinary care teams, and work with caregivers to implement survivorship plans that center whole-person care. (Bader, Graham, Mbayo, Pivor)

Reducing financial barriers to equitable care
- Develop, test, and disseminate financial models that sustainably support survivorship, wellness, and recovery care. (Alfano, Brasfield, Reid)
- Enhance and expand access to health insurance and reduce costs for patients through measures such as expanding Medicaid eligibility, reducing administrative barriers, enhancing subsidies for insurance purchased through the marketplace, reviewing plans to ensure adequate network and team care coverage, and lowering annual out-of-pocket caps. (Dusetzina, Rosenbaum, Perkins)
- Use value-based payment models, such as the Enhancing Oncology Model, and improve policies to reimburse for team care. (Cavanagh, Dusetzina)
- Incorporate time-based billing to account for various clinician tasks, including care outside the day of service. (Choi)

BOX 2 Continued

Expanding advocacy and investment
- Identify health equity issues and advocate for legislation, policies, and interventions to address them. (Fuld Nasso)
- Recognize care inequities as a human rights issue and spur investment in building dedicated programs to address disparities. (Allicock, Fuld Nasso, Irwin, Ma)

Focusing on patient perspectives and needs
- Listen to patient feedback and couple patient-reported outcomes with clinical measures. (Allicock, Cavanagh, Stout)
- Redesign follow-up visits to center patients' needs, include self-management strategies, and relieve high clinical workload. (Mayer)

Enhancing survivorship care
- Prioritize and fund research on survivorship care that promotes health equity and centers patient and caregiver experiences. (Tonorezos)
- Develop and disseminate guidelines for care transitions and examine standards, curricula, and licensure requirements to improve survivorship care. (Mayer, Shulman)
- Develop high-quality, multidisciplinary survivorship care models for cancer center accreditation and evaluation. (Shulman, Yabroff)
- Initiate care planning at diagnosis and use a billing code for patient navigation. (Fuld Nasso)
- Train and support clinicians and navigators who focus specifically on survivorship. (Choi, Fuld Nasso, Jacobs, Malin, Pirl, Winn)

NOTE: This list is the rapporteurs' synopsis of observations made by one or more individual speakers as identified. These statements have not been endorsed or verified by the National Academies of Sciences, Engineering, and Medicine. They are not intended to reflect a consensus among workshop participants.

BOX 3
Experiences Shared by Cancer Survivors

Several speakers emphasized that a systems-level view is important for making lasting improvements in cancer and survivorship care but noted that it is ultimately the needs of the patients that drive the necessity for these improvements. To ground the workshop discussions in the needs and priorities of people with cancer, several cancer survivors shared perspectives on their care experiences.

After she was diagnosed with endometrial cancer in 2017, Jacqueline Mbayo, director of research partnerships at the Endometrial Cancer Action Network for African Americans (ECANA), said that she received excellent care from her team, which included a gynecologist, gynecologic oncologist, medical oncologist, radiation oncologist, primary care physician (PCP), social workers, multiple nurses and technicians, and caregivers. These team members addressed treatment barriers and side effects, communicated and coordinated with her and each other, and encouraged her to advocate for her treatment, survival, and quality-of-life needs. In contrast, Mbayo noted that in her work at ECANA, she often hears stories of people who are misdiagnosed, dismissed, or receive poor care. She said that it is her mission to ensure that everyone receives the same extraordinary care that she did.

Susan Bader has had multiple cancers and treatment-related lung and heart complications. For much of her decades-long cancer journey, she said that she felt alone and unsupported. More recently, she has begun to feel more confident with a survivorship plan, a trusted primary care clinician, and a team of specialists who understand and address her multiple, layered health issues. In her view, the two most critical improvements needed in cancer care are to implement survivorship plans and include primary care clinicians on the care team and in every decision, from diagnosis to posttreatment.

Alia Graham, founder and president of Head Up, Inc., reflected on her experience with triple-negative breast cancer, a type of breast cancer that has a very poor prognosis. She shared that in the beginning, her treatment experience was so poor that she decided to seek care at a different hospital. The second hospital provided much higher-quality care from a more empathetic team, and while the course of treatment was very physically and mentally difficult, she credits her recovery to not only this team but also her self-advocacy, positivity, and determination to seek out true helpers.

> **BOX 3 Continued**
>
> While she initially feared she would not survive her disease, she has now been cancer free for 3 years.
>
> Jeremy Pivor, senior program coordinator of Planetary Health Alliance at Harvard University, was first diagnosed with cancer at age 12. During this first cancer experience, he had access to multidisciplinary team care, which is common in pediatric cancer. In treatment for recurrences during adulthood, however, he has found the care to be very different. Instead of being set up with a team designed to provide "whole-person care," he said that he had to essentially assemble one himself, which has been a time-intensive, laborious task requiring strong self-advocacy. He said that having such a team is critical to providing patients with guidance on what to expect, alleviating some of their logistical stress, and removing treatment barriers. The team care approach also helps specialists to connect with patients' humanity and psychosocial needs.
>
> Anita Gupta, adjunct assistant professor at Johns Hopkins University, is both a clinician and a cancer survivor. She shared that her experience as a patient with cancer—one with the access and know-how to navigate the system and get the very best care—shed light on inequitable access to care, discrimination, and the lack of empathy many patients face. She recalled feeling like some clinicians saw her as merely a patient in a gown and not a whole person with a family, a career, her own expertise, and a unique set of hopes and dreams. She stressed that equitable access to multidisciplinary care is only possible if clinicians feel a deep compassion for their patients as people and a sense of purpose in their work. She observed that public health is a humanitarian issue, and a concerted, collaborative approach is crucial to addressing the human needs that are at the center of a patient's health priorities.
>
> SOURCES: Patient perspectives video presentations and Anita Gupta presentation, July 17, 2023.

of nursing and founding director of the cancer survivorship program at the University of Pennsylvania Abramson Cancer Center (ACS, 2023).

Jacobs noted that at each stage of the cancer treatment and survivorship continuum—from diagnosis and treatment to rehabilitation and survivorship—patients have very different needs, concerns, and challenges that affect their relationships with their caregivers, oncologists, and other specialists. Carlson and Jacobs pointed out that problems can mount over time and comorbidities become more common with age. Moreover, the challenges of survivorship care grow more complex as an increasing number of cancer survivors live for decades past their diagnosis and often well into old age (see Figure 1) (ASCO, 2020; Bluethmann et al., 2016; Miller et al., 2022).

As the number of aging cancer survivors grows, it becomes increasingly difficult for health systems to keep pace with patient needs, said Deborah K. Mayer, Francis Hill Fox distinguished professor emeritus at the University of North Carolina at Chapel Hill School of Nursing (Bluethmann et al., 2016; Mariotto et al., 2022). She observed that there is often a disconnect between patient and clinician perspectives on care following cancer treatment. At most follow-up appointments, clinicians are mainly looking for tumor recurrence, while patients are often concerned about quality-of-life considerations, such as exercise, nutrition, and physical and mental function. To make these visits more meaningful, Mayer emphasized that patients need to be asked the right questions by clinicians who understand patient priorities.

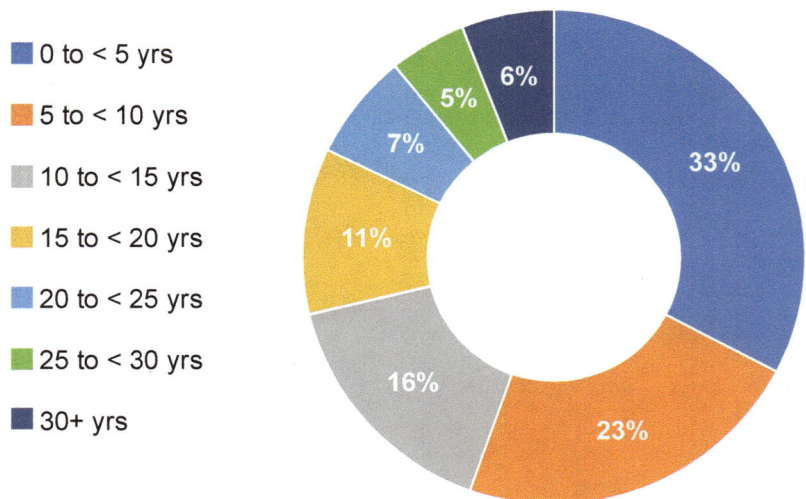

FIGURE 1 U.S. cancer survivors by years from diagnosis.
SOURCES: Carlson presentation, July 17, 2023; ACS, 2019.

Mayer suggested that clinicians need to think differently about the many subpopulations of cancer survivors and create flexible systems that are more adaptable to each patient's needs. She pointed out that the groundwork for such a system was outlined in a 2006 Institute of Medicine report, but its vision has not been realized, and the current clinical workforce is not equipped to fill the existing gaps (IOM and NRC, 2006). She added that despite the enormous number of clinical appointments cancer survivors typically attend—incurring both time and resource burdens on patients and health systems—little evidence exists on the effectiveness of different follow-up strategies on outcomes such as overall survival, quality of life, and time to recurrence (Chan et al., 2023; Høeg et al., 2019). Mayer described the current situation as a "free-for-all," with clinics struggling to meet the high volume of patients and yet unsure about the benefits of all these appointments. "The current way we do it isn't really working very well, but we are very busy doing it," Mayer said. "We really need to think about that, and with every visit, we need to be asking ourselves, 'Is this the best thing for this patient?'"

The Role of Specialty Care and the Need for Coordination

Because many cancer survivors face a range of long-term health issues related to their cancer and cancer treatment, they often require care involving many medical specialties, from reproductive health and fertility to endocrinology and cardiology, and dozens of other areas. For example, Jeremy Pivor, senior program coordinator of Planetary Health Alliance at Harvard University, said that his care requires a large multispecialty and multidisciplinary team including expertise from primary care, cardiology, medical and radiation oncology, physical therapy, occupational therapy, psychiatry, acupuncture, neurosurgery, rheumatology, neurology, and a therapist who specializes in treating young adults with cancer (see Box 3).

Carlson pointed out that the number of cancer survivors is growing much more rapidly than the number of specialists. Even medical centers that have a good mix of specialists face challenges integrating them into a functional, collaborative care team focused on survivorship, said Jacobs. She highlighted a number of common challenges, including:

- lack of survivorship-focused education and training for the health care workforce, especially for non-oncologists;
- difficulties in coordinating referrals and long-term follow-ups with clinicians; and
- addressing geographic and financial barriers for patients to access appropriate care.

Carlson and Jacobs also noted that the frequent disconnect in how people think about the timeline of survivorship care: cancer treatment centers are accustomed to discharging patients from follow-up care after 5 years, yet patients require personalized care that is responsive to their evolving needs throughout the lifespan.

As an example, Jacobs described a patient who received treatment in 1994 for Hodgkin lymphoma. This patient had very few health problems until she experienced thyroid failure in 2012, followed closely by breast lymphoma, sinus tachycardia, and other serious health issues over the ensuing decade, including esophageal cancer, and most recently aortic stenosis requiring surgical intervention. Her care team is multidisciplinary, yet she still struggles to find specialized care for her myriad issues. In complex situations like these, Jacobs noted the little guidance available to aid decision making, expand or consolidate care, and incorporate new therapies.

The transition from pediatric cancer treatment and survivorship care to adult care can pose special challenges, as outlined by Lillian Meacham, professor of pediatrics at Emory University and director of the Fertility Preservation and Reproductive Health Program at Children's Healthcare of Atlanta. She described the difficulty her pediatric patients had in accessing long-term survivorship visits until she began framing them as essential care. Jacobs related that her center's survivorship program began as a partnership with the Children's Hospital of Pennsylvania's (CHOP) late-effects clinic. Although the relationship started slowly because the two centers are so different, over time they have developed an important foundation of trust, and CHOP clinicians now feel more confident sending patients to her center for survivorship care as they transition into adult care.

To delve deeper into some of the common health issues survivors face, the need for specialty care, and potential opportunities to enhance care coordination, many speakers shared experiences and models from the perspective of a range of medical specializations. While not comprehensively inclusive of the full spectrum of areas relevant to cancer survivorship care, speakers discussed a sampling of approaches to enhance multidisciplinary, multispecialty care.

Cardio-oncology

Cardiovascular disease (CVD) and cancer are two of the leading causes of death worldwide, and the prevalence of both conditions is growing, said Bonnie Ky, Founders associate professor of cardio-oncology at the University of Pennsylvania (Global Burden of Disease 2019 Cancer Collaboration, 2022; Roth et al., 2020). Ky noted that cardio-oncology, a specialization that bridges these disease types, is well positioned to provide evidence-based, empathetic, accessible, inclusive care. Improvements in cancer diagnosis, treatment, and management have contributed in part to the growing number of people living with and beyond cancer, but many face an elevated risk of CVD, often as a result of the cardiotoxic effects of cancer treatments (Armenian et al., 2016; Chow et al., 2022; Gallicchio et al., 2022; Miller et al., 2022). Ky observed that despite this known risk, which increases with age, many cancer survivors with CVD are underdiagnosed and undertreated and face a higher risk of death than the general population (Paterson et al., 2022; Strongman et al., 2022; Sun et al., 2021). Similarly, patients with CVD are often diagnosed with cancer and have an increased risk of cancer mortality (Bell et al., 2023; Bertero et al., 2022).

Ky outlined a conceptual model with potential strategies for equitable, evidence-based care to enable patients with cancer to live longer, healthier lives (see Figure 2). First, she highlighted the importance of developing, evaluating, and adopting practice- and system-level inclusive, evidence-based, collaborative care delivery models. She noted that these should be patient centered; define and equip gatekeepers, hubs, and spokes; emphasize communication; include support layers; and leverage scalable technologies and findings from behavioral economics research (Adusumalli et al., 2023; Demissei et al., 2020; Waddell et al., 2020; Zullig et al., 2021).

Second, Ky called for further investment to advance precision CVD risk phenotyping and reduction throughout the lifespan, noting that such advancements will require more detailed, integrated, multi-omics and machine learning (ML) phenotyping methods to better identify and aid patients who may be at a high risk for developing CVD; a more modern, epidemiological definition of CVD, and cardio-protection targeting and treatment strategies (Armenian et al., 2016). Additionally, a better understanding of the basic biology of CVD and cancer needs to be translated into effective treatments to improve care and patient outcomes.

Third, Ky urged the community to prioritize mitigating disparities in CVD outcomes by recognizing and addressing geographical and race-based inequities in care (Noyd et al., 2023; Tsui et al., 2020; Zhu et al., 2023). Specifically, she noted a need for more research to examine CVD risk by ancestry and understand the social determinants of health (SDOH) at the intersection of CVD and cancer. She added that it is imperative to enhance diversity in clinical trials and to incorporate equity, accessibility, and partnerships with community health centers (CHCs) to ensure patient- and community-centered care (Johnson, 2023).

Finally, Ky stressed that future workforce training should prioritize effective, empathic, and resilient care; rigorous science and patient-centered practices; and clinical and scientific training (Alvarez-Cardona et al., 2020; Tuzovic et al., 2020). She noted that this will require developing new training standards and metrics, investing in and incentivizing early-career researchers, addressing

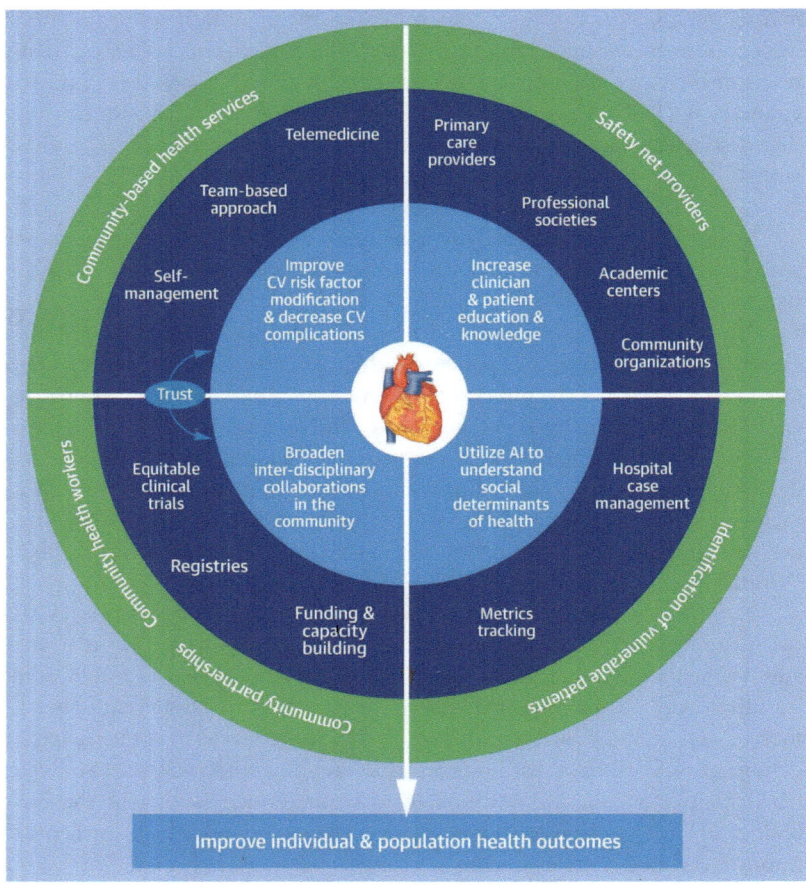

FIGURE 2 Strategies to mitigate inequities and disparities at the intersection of cardiovascular disease and cancer.
NOTE: AI = artificial intelligence; CV = cardiovascular.
SOURCES: Ky presentation, July 17, 2023; Johnson, 2023, CC BY NC ND 4.0.

workforce stressors, and establishing formal, multidisciplinary, multiorganizational collaborations (Shulman et al., 2020; Takvorian et al., 2020).

Rehabilitation Medicine

Rehabilitative care models that are co-located and embedded with cancer care delivery can play a crucial role in addressing the high burden of post-cancer disability, noted Nicole Stout, associate director of the survivorship program at West Virginia University. Although these models have been well known for some time and applied to many other medical specialties, they have only recently been effectively adopted in cancer care, and only in a few settings, she said.

Embedded rehabilitative care can take different forms, she explained, but it is always supported and informed by patient-reported outcomes (PROs) and integrated into clinical workflows. Such care is based on the Prospective Surveillance Model of repeated screening, identification of functional deficits, need stratification, and determination of next care steps (Stout et al., 2012). Stout noted that features of this care model may also be billable through the Centers for Medicare & Medicaid Services (CMS), which is an important consideration for health systems.

Stout detailed several real-world examples of embedded rehabilitative care:

- In a study from the University of Utah, a physical therapist (PT) embedded in a thoracic oncology center provides repeated precision exercise prescriptions for patients with lung cancer that are adapted in response to changes in a patient's functioning (Barnes et al., 2020; Ulrich et al., 2018).
- At the West Virginia University Cancer Institute Brain Tumor Clinic, embedded occupational therapists see patients in tandem with neuro-oncologists to determine next care steps and navigate referrals (Stout et al., 2023a).
- In reports from two cancer center clinical service lines in Florida, PTs also serve as patient navigators, assessing function and coordinating appropriate care (Stout et al., 2023b; Stout et al., 2019).

Stout observed that patients report greater satisfaction with their treatment when their needs are more fully addressed through such care models (Stout et al., 2023b). She attributed the success of these models to the fact that they were implemented within cancer care, were aligned with systemwide strategies, and had a high level of institutional support.

Stout also noted that rehabilitative care can be better integrated into existing care systems by embedding processes and algorithms into electronic health records (EHRs) to proactively screen and identify patients in need of services or referrals. She shared one example in which the use of such an approach with an "opt-out" model was shown to reduce physician burden and increase patient use of supportive services (Stout et al., 2023c). In another example, of a technology-driven rehabilitation model at the Mayo Clinic, oncology PTs remotely coach generalist PTs on caring for patients with cancer, resulting in decreased hospital utilization and improved use of outpatient care (Cheville et al., 2018, 2019).

Stout observed that the team approach to patient care is redefining cancer survivorship (Alfano et al., 2022), but she said that further work is needed to

- achieve standardized, function-driven care via assessments and tools that couple PROs with clinical measures;
- advance research on embedded rehabilitation;
- develop shared, aligned rehab-oncology services;
- optimize the cancer care capacities of PTs through education and knowledge translation; and
- provide payment incentives for more comprehensive survivorship services.

Psychosocial Health

Gaps in the provision of mental health care and the role of psychosocial health in collaborative cancer care were discussed by William Pirl, vice chair for psychosocial oncology at Dana-Farber Cancer Institute, and Kelly Irwin, director of the Collaborative Care and Community Engagement Program at Massachusetts General Hospital Cancer Center. They explained that psychosocial health affects every aspect of life, including mental health, physical functioning, finances, and even mortality. Pirl said that the shortage of U.S. mental health care clinicians—an estimated 30 million people with mental illness are not receiving services or face long wait times—underscores the challenge and importance of proactive steps to incorporate psychosocial health into cancer care (Beck et al., 2018; Hewitt and Rowland, 2002; HRSA, 2023a). Irwin noted that mental health care has far fewer resources, is far less accessible, and is far more fragmented than cancer care. As a result, many patients with mental health conditions are undertreated, socially isolated, and at higher risk of experiencing homelessness. Moreover, oncologists lack training to care for patients with complex mental health diagnoses. Irwin added that people with mental health disorders are frequently discriminated against and systematically excluded from clinical trials (Humphreys et al., 2015; Irwin et al., 2019).

These factors result in poor outcomes for patients with both cancer and mental illness, who suffer disparities in cancer prevention, screening, diagnosis, treatment selection, palliative care referrals, and mortality (Irwin et al., 2014). Stressing the need for a strong, collaborative network to advocate for the care needs of people with mental illness, Irwin said that "if we don't do this, we're saying that these peoples' lives have less value than other people's lives."

Although most cancer centers offer general psychosocial care, Pirl explained that many patients need more specialized care, such as from social workers, psychologists, or psychiatrists (Deshields et al., 2013). The referral process is complicated with long wait times because frequent follow-ups are necessary and because clinicians prioritize current patients. Telehealth has alleviated some access barriers, such as geographic maldistribution of clinicians and inability of patients to travel for care, but access is still limited by the number of clinicians, Pirl noted.

Pirl offered a few guiding principles for improving psychosocial health as part of collaborative cancer care. He said there will never be adequate numbers of mental health clinicians, so it is essential to integrate mental health care within medical care. He pointed out that behavioral therapy is often as effective as medication for many conditions; a stepped-care approach[4] can support efficient use of resources; and screening and tracking are essential to ensuring patient populations are receiving adequate and evidence-based care. Moreover, including a care manager who coordinates mental health care can facilitate truly collaborative care. Pirl said studies have shown that patients receiving collaborative care reported improvements in anxiety, depression, functioning, and quality of life (Ell et al., 2008; Kroenke et al., 2010; Walker et al., 2014).

Pirl noted that collaborative care is evidence based, CMS supported, consistent with ASCO guidelines, and can be effectively implemented in cancer clinics, where staff are often already trained to assess psychosocial needs and make referrals (Pirl et al., 2020; Tsao et al., 2023; Wu et al., 2023). It is also scalable through integration of remote and onsite workers; shared, flexible, unified workflows for evaluation, screening, care, and follow-up; and coordination with local community resources and mental health clinicians. Collaborative care has not yet become well known or widely adopted outside of primary care, which Pirl attributed to the perceived effort required for implementation. He emphasized the growing momentum to train the workforce to deliver psychosocial collaborative care in oncology.

Palliative Care

Palliative care is an example of a field that has successfully implemented team-based care, said Arif Kamal, chief patient officer at the American Cancer Society. With its focus on both the short- and long-term needs of patients and their caregivers, as a unit, at every stage along the cancer continuum and a commitment to promote patients' and caregivers' stated priorities regarding both quality and quantity of life, palliative care is fundamentally multidisciplinary, multispecialty, and team based, he explained. He added that it is naturally team based because the drivers of patient and caregiver suffering—physical, emotional, and financial—are too interconnected and complex for one clinician to address. Serious illness care has evolved over time, Kamal

---

[4] The stepped-care model includes four steps: watchful waiting, self-help psychotherapy, face-to-face psychotherapy, and referral to specialists (Ho et al., 2016).

said, and patients are now receiving care in multiple settings and increasingly at home. Care is also spanning longer timeframes, with a heightened focus on health-related social needs and greater recognition of caregivers' needs.

Kamal noted that quality measurement frameworks for palliative care can be integrated into oncology to deliver effective care whether a patient has a chronic, stable disease state, has progressive disease, or is nearing the end of life (NQF, 2006).

Kamal said the number of quality palliative care training programs is growing, including those offering advanced degrees, certifications, and mid-career fellowships (Kamal et al., 2015, 2016). However, although the field has grown rapidly, he said that palliative care is not uniformly available across the United States: There is a widespread workforce shortage, and reimbursement can be challenging (Heitner et al., 2019; Kamal et al., 2019). He also cautioned that patients will not benefit equally until other factors that affect patient outcomes can be addressed, such as a lack of transportation, gaps in health or digital literacy, and the high cost of cancer care.

Kamal pointed to several examples of draft legislation before Congress that aim to improve patient care by funding needed training, attracting more diverse patients into clinical trials, and enabling social workers to bill for health-related social services currently considered outside their scope of practice. In addition, Kamal noted that the White House is expected to announce that patient navigation, even by community health workers and nonprofessionals, will be covered by Medicare. "This is a nice tidal wave going in the right direction," Kamal said. However, without these changes, he warned that there is a risk that the increased need for team-based care that integrates palliative specialists will go unmet.

Primary Care

Primary care physicians are well equipped to handle many issues on the continuum of cancer care, such as comorbidity, preventive care, cancer screening, and referral management, observed Youngjee Choi, assistant professor of medicine at Johns Hopkins University. However, despite good models for integrating primary care into cancer care, most clinicians find themselves in a shared-care model that is unintentional, lacks effective communication, and creates gaps and redundancies (Nekhlyudov et al., 2017). She said that risk stratification workflows are needed to determine a patient's risk category and assign or share care (Figure 3). Choi added that primary care providers (PCPs) and oncologists need to clarify their roles and designate responsibilities. She also suggested that professional organizations should collaborate on developing readily accessible risk stratification guidelines or algorithms.

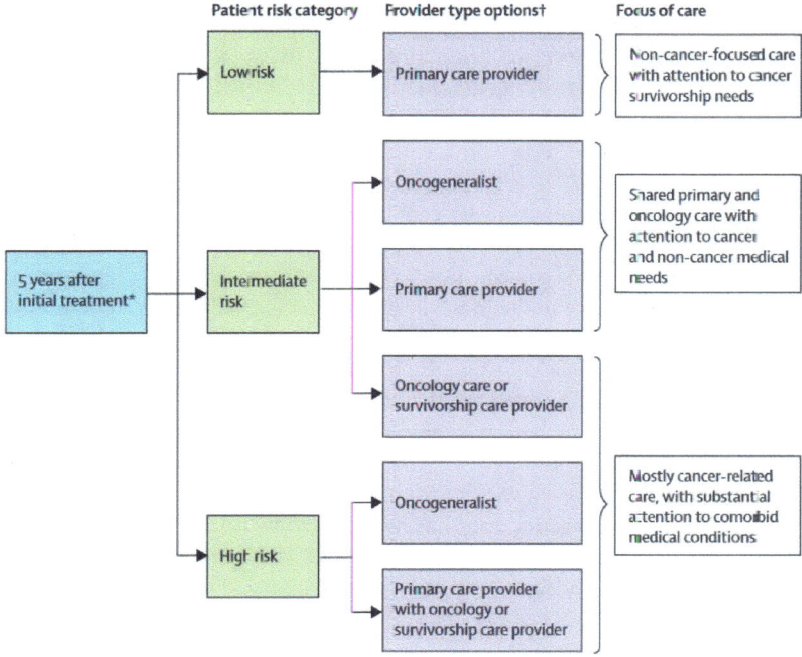

FIGURE 3 An example risk stratification workflow for cancer survivorship care. SOURCES: Choi presentation, July 17, 2023; Nekhlyudov et al., 2017. Reprinted from *Lancet Oncology*, 18(1), Nekhlyudov, L., D. M. O'Malley, and S. V. Hudson. Integrating primary care providers in the care of cancer survivors: Gaps in evidence and future opportunities, e30-e38, 2017, with permission from Elsevier.

Reproductive Health and Fertility

Undergoing cancer treatments in childhood or young adulthood can involve significant reproductive risks. Clarisa Gracia, chief of reproductive endocrinology and infertility at the University of Pennsylvania, stressed that it is crucial for clinicians to inform patients about these risks as soon as possible and ensure that patients and their families are aware of fertility preservation options, which have greatly improved in recent years. Providing access to reproductive care and counseling is important to support the individual's well-being and long-term health, she said. However, she noted that referrals to reproductive health specialists can have long wait times and high costs, posing equity concerns, and fertility preservation interventions can require extra travel and treatment delays.

Endocrinology

Describing the role of endocrinologists in cancer survivorship care, Meacham pointed out that the endocrine system is easily damaged by cancer therapies, which can cause problems that greatly diminish patients' quality of life. Such problems, however, are often diagnosed too late (Hudson et al., 2013; Pradhan et al., 2019). Meacham explained that many patients face barriers in accessing this specialty care due to cost, time, hesitancy to see yet another clinician, and limited availability of subspecialists in certain areas.

Meacham pointed to the need for exposure-focused, evidence-based, long-term surveillance guidelines, noting that it is challenging to determine who is responsible for this surveillance, especially as pediatric patients transition to adult care. To help bridge the gap and enable more patients to access care, she suggested that oncology clinicians could be provided with short summaries highlighting key late endocrine effects of cancer treatments to encourage better surveillance and that survivors could also receive more information to help them drive their own follow-up care. She referred to Project ECHO[5] as an informative resource for sharing best practices and knowledge with communities that are rural and/or underserved, while providing specialty care when facilities lack endocrinologists or other experts.

Pulmonology

Including pulmonologists as a part of multidisciplinary cancer care teams can improve patient outcomes in several ways, explained Patrick Nana-Sinkam, professor of medicine at Virginia Commonwealth University. During and after cancer treatment, pulmonologists can help address complications from therapy, which can include pneumonia and other lung problems. Across the care continuum, they can inform decisions about screening to diagnose lung cancer and other lung or arterial diseases, such as chronic obstructive pulmonary disease, a lethal disease that is frequently underdiagnosed or mismanaged (Deepak et al., 2015; Gaga et al., 2013). Pulmonary specialists can also integrate tobacco cessation, physical therapy, disease stage–specific care, interventional pulmonology tools, and mutational screening algorithms into a patient's cancer treatment and survivorship care, he noted.

---

[5] See https://www.ahrq.gov/patient-safety/settings/multiple/project-echo/index.html (accessed December 29, 2023).

Nutrition

Malnutrition is common among cancer survivors and leads to adverse outcomes, said Cynthia Thomson, professor of health promotion sciences at University of Arizona (NIH, 2023; Ryan et al., 2016; Thompson et al., 2017). She noted that effective assessment tools exist and survivors are often open to supportive nutrition care. Many organizations are working to disseminate evidence-based guidance (Arends et al., 2017), but barriers have hindered full integration into cancer survivorship, including a dearth of nutritionists in some areas, limited specialized training in nutri-oncology, a lack of reimbursement for medical nutritional therapy, and low funding for nutri-oncology research (Trujillo et al., 2019). As a result, nutritional management is often crisis management. To better support patients and survivors, Thomson stressed that nutrition care should be integrated into patient-centered screening tools and EHRs, delivered via telehealth, recognized as an evidence-based specialty reimbursable by insurers and CMS, more widely shared with patients to combat misinformation, and supported with more research funding (Bossi et al., 2021; Eisman et al., 2021; Prado et al., 2022). She also suggested that future efforts focus on assessing the cost effectiveness of nutrition care, expanding research into more diverse populations, creating a national multidisciplinary guideline for nutrition therapy, and developing a standard of care for screening and assessment.

Cognition

The majority of patients report cancer-related cognitive impairments, said Diane Von Ah, distinguished professor at The Ohio State University College of Nursing. The most common are related to memory and executive function, and approximately one-third of patients experience clinically significant deficits. She said that these cancer-related cognitive impairments have a large impact on patients' quality of life, mental ability, physical functioning, and mortality (Lange et al., 2019). They are complex and appear throughout the cancer survivorship continuum, often co-occurring with other symptoms. She explained that they can be affected by cancer treatments and various SDOH.

Von Ah noted that despite the prevalence of these cognitive impairments, interventions are limited, and there are few clinical guidelines. She underscored the need for multidisciplinary, multispecialty care and coordination to implement valid and reliable assessments for identifying cognitive impairments across all age groups, use better diagnostic tools for correlating symptoms and provide referrals for care in a way that does not burden patients. Von Ah emphasized that more research and increased workforce training is essential.

Coordination Roles

Many speakers throughout the workshop discussed the importance of having people specifically dedicated to coordinating care. Choi suggested that social workers can be helpful for care coordination. Catherine Alfano, vice president of cancer care management and research at Northwell Health, stated that risk and needs stratification, which benefits the patient, can also reduce clinicians' time and patient load. She described how Northwell created a new position for taking a comprehensive view of the patient and bringing in specialists as needed, in an effort to use teams more efficiently. Shulman added that dedicated survivorship clinics are also able to take a more long-term perspective, looking for downstream cancer and treatment effects, managing them, and referring patients to specialists as needed.

Addressing Disparities

Winn said that more than 30 million people living in the United States, many from historically underserved populations, receive their medical care at federally qualified health centers (FQHCs), also known as community health centers (CHCs) (HSRA, 2023b). Sidney and Emily Kark opened the first CHC in South Africa in 1942, to provide care as well as training for local doctors and nurses and education for the public on health practices (Tollman, 1994). After meeting the Karks in the 1960s, Jack Geiger, Count Gibson, and John Hatch opened the first U.S. CHCs with a focus on overcoming social injustices.[6] There are now more than 15,000 CHCs across the United States delivering multidisciplinary integrated care.[7] Many also employ lay health advisors—trained community members who promote and protect health while addressing the unequal burden of cancer and other diseases in communities that have been historically marginalized.

Winn said that CHCs are not being used to their full potential to provide care and reduce disparities in the context of cancer and survivorship care. He stressed that although it can be tempting to focus on the latest treatment advances that could offer slightly better survival rates, attending to essential care needs is crucial. He cautioned against losing sight of the imperative to ensure that people get the treatments they need. He posited that CHCs could take a much bigger role in this, saying "we have a tool that was supposed to

---

[6] See https://geigergibson.publichealth.gwu.edu/geiger-and-gibson (accessed December 29, 2023).

[7] See https://www.nachc.org/resource/americas-health-centers-by-the-numbers/ (accessed April 18, 2024).

be the undergirding in the United States for our most vulnerable, and we have in some ways ignored what was put in place."

Describing his work to incorporate research, specialist care, and survivorship into a Chicago FQHC's traditional care model and public health focus, Winn said that academic cancer centers and CHCs should collaborate on aligning their communities, programs, services, and strategic directions to achieve greater equity in cancer and survivorship care. Both types of centers also need to acknowledge the social drivers of health affecting patient outcomes, which operate across the institutional, neighborhood, and biological spectra. Finally, Winn stressed that CHCs need "activators" who, instead of merely navigating health services (which sometimes fall short), actually advocate for their patients' needs.

Reflecting on Winn's comments, Gwen Darien, the executive vice president of patient advocacy and engagement at the National Patient Advocate Foundation, said that it is critical to avoid inadvertently exacerbating inequities when developing systems for multidisciplinary, multispecialty care. Winn said that addressing inequities is difficult, but if the cancer community can overcome the challenges involved in developing novel therapies, there is no reason why the same sort of effort could not be applied to overcoming inequities in care. Furthermore, there are known solutions that could make significant progress toward revolutionizing community health care and improve lives with little difficulty or cost, such as hiring trusted community activators, Winn said. Darien echoed this point, reiterating that most patients are treated in their communities, not at large centers.

Jacobs said that many CHC clinicians feel they lack the expertise to treat patients with cancer, and she suggested that additional education could help them feel more comfortable managing the care of patients with complex conditions. Because many CHCs do not have oncologists on staff, another participant suggested that cancer centers could partner with CHCs to improve their scope of practice and handle more survivorship care in these settings.

Advancing Multidisciplinary, Multispecialty Care

Many speakers highlighted a variety of approaches that could be leveraged to help facilitate multidisciplinary, multispecialty care. Mayer offered several suggestions for improving survivorship care at the patient level, including better care communication, coordination, and facilitation; more effective efforts to remove barriers to care; and research evaluating different care models. She also suggested that follow-up visits need to be redesigned to center on a patient's needs, include self-management strategies, and relieve the high clinical volume. To address these issues at a systems level, Mayer underscored the need for NCCN guidelines for care transitions. She also suggested that federal agencies, professional associations, and health systems need to collaboratively examine standards, identify gaps, develop curricula and licensure requirements, create incentives, pool resources, improve recruitment and retention, and design self-management and advocacy tools for different populations.

Mayer emphasized that more workers are needed, in all fields, in all areas of the country, and from all backgrounds, to fill workforce gaps and address disparities in access, care, and outcomes (Perlmutter et al., 2022; Shih et al., 2021). However, staffing shortages are not likely to be easily resolved, noted Amye Tevaarwerk, oncologist at the Mayo Clinic and practice chair for the Division of Medical Oncology in Rochester. To increase the efficiency and effectiveness of the existing workforce, she said that clinicians could benefit from better leveraging tools and technology. "None of us can work harder—we have to work smarter," she said. Mayer suggested that it may be possible to harness new technologies, such as ML and artificial intelligence (AI), to "work smarter" on patient-centered care that streamlines visits with multiple clinicians, screens for unmet needs and ongoing problems more effectively, and tailors care to each situation.

Shulman pointed out that medicine has been slow to adopt digital opportunities that can make care more efficient, especially when patients require the care of multiple specialists. Pirl noted that PROs can be helpful if patients fill them out over time, and that natural language processing (NLP) technologies are now robust enough to be integrated into EHRs to screen for needs and coordinate care. One caveat, Winn pointed out, is that NLP and similar techniques require quality data, but current data sources often leave out entire communities and millions of people, especially those who visit CHCs and may have unique needs. Shulman agreed that this is an important consideration and noted that many AI protocols are now integrating human elements to address such data gaps and disparities.

Douglas Peterson, head of oral medicine at University of Connecticut Health, cautioned that the inability of patients to adhere to treatment regimens can pose a challenge to ensuring high-quality care even with the most dedicated health care team. Shulman agreed, noting that researchers are investigating technologies to increase adherence. Winn pointed out that technology alone is not enough and that high-touch practices are also needed. Stout agreed, adding that her patients in rural West Virginia do not readily adopt new technologies. She explained that although technological advances would be welcome to help West Virginia's underfunded CHCs integrate their EHR data, the real need is for PCPs and CHCs to have a better understanding of cancer care and navigation, and to better help patients optimize self-management skills and overcome negative health beliefs, she said (Azriful et al., 2021).

EDUCATION AND TRAINING OPPORTUNITIES

Several speakers stressed that most clinicians do not receive the training they need to sustainably implement multidisciplinary, multispecialty collaborative care in practice. Multiple speakers explored ways to transition from a clinic-by-clinic or program-by-program strategy to facilitate broader changes. They discussed potential collaborative educational frameworks and opportunities to integrate collaborative care models into education, training, and practice.

Mayer and Jacobs stressed that the current education and training infrastructure supporting both patients and clinicians is inadequate. Mayer explained that staff at all levels need more training and more effective partnerships. Jacobs pointed out that the current educational pipeline is insufficient to create the multidisciplinary, multispecialty workforce that is needed. Nekhlyudov observed that improving survivorship care should start with oncologists themselves—many of whom lack a deep understanding of what such comprehensive care entails—before moving into more widespread workforce training. Carlson agreed but added that overworked oncology practices and nursing shortages pose significant challenges and may make it difficult for many oncologists to take on additional training. Winn suggested that survivorship should be seen as an integral part of care rather than segmenting "survivorship" clinicians. He urged a focus on creating more oncology generalists who can focus on aligning survivorship care.

Choi suggested that enhancing cancer survivorship education earlier—in medical school and during residencies—could help to address many of the gaps in care delivery and coordination. She said this would be especially important for CHC clinicians and PCPs who may not have access to academic institutions or cancer centers. Gracia agreed and noted that cancer survivorship has been integrated into reproductive fellowships. Ky added that professional societies are working to improve workforce and community education, but it is challenging to implement these strategies, especially for those most in need.

Interprofessional Collaborative Practice and Interprofessional Education

Mitchell Heflin, professor of medicine in the Division of Geriatrics at Duke University Schools of Nursing and Medicine, and Sallie Weaver, a senior scientist and program director in the Health Systems and Interventions Research Branch at the National Cancer Institute (NCI), discussed how interprofessional collaborative practice (IPCP) and interprofessional education

(IPE)[8] can improve patient care by creating a collaboration-ready, multidisciplinary cancer care workforce that can equitably deliver the increasingly complex, comprehensive health services that patients, caregivers, and communities need (IOM, 2008, 2013).

Heflin noted that cancer care services are becoming increasingly interdisciplinary, especially in light of efforts to address the SDOH. Effective teamwork is essential to achieve health goals, deliver optimal care, eliminate inequities, and optimize the workforce (Greilich et al., 2023; Salas et al., 2009; Tannenbaum et al., 2021). He added that although graduates in the health professions are clinically competent, their lack of IPE and IPCP preparation contributes to errors, low clinician and patient satisfaction, system inefficiencies, and higher costs (IOM, 2000, 2015).

Heflin and Weaver explained that IPE and IPCP emphasize co-education, collaboration, and interaction. Effective IPCP team members share expertise, ideas, and decision making with humility and mutual respect; have flexible leadership but defined roles; employ clear communication; question assumptions and hierarchies; and work toward shared goals (Spaulding et al., 2021; Weaver et al., 2018). Studies indicate that this type of teamwork results in more affordable and accessible care, better care adherence, fewer errors and readmissions, shorter hospital stays, and greater patient and clinician satisfaction, Heflin said (Babiker et al., 2014; McDonald et al., 2018; McGuier et al., 2021; Reeves et al., 2016).

The core competencies and characteristics of IPE/IPCP focus on patient-, family-, community-, and population-centered approaches and concern the entire spectrum of learning, licensure, and practice. Weaver said that competency domains of team-based care include patient-centered care, communication, shared mental models, and coordination (Chollette et al., 2020). Heflin and Weaver said that implementation is necessary at various levels, including patient care, clinician practices, leadership, education, policy, administration, and within academic–CHC clinical partnerships (Bogossian et al., 2023; IPEC, 2016).

Challenges to implementing IPE and IPCP include a lack of reimbursement or other funding mechanisms, a lack of functioning models in clinical practice, inadequate education and training, and a general resistance to change, Heflin said. Weaver described how an IPE curriculum that emphasizes critical and clearly defined teamwork competencies can not only improve patient care

---

[8] Interprofessional education occurs when two or more professions learn about, from, and with each other to enable effective collaboration and improve health outcomes, while interprofessional collaborative practice occurs when multiple health workers from different professional backgrounds provide comprehensive health services by working with patients, their families, carers, and communities to deliver the highest quality of care (Gilbert et al., 2010).

and practice efficiency but also prepare clinicians to be competent members of their immediate team and of a larger constellation of teams (see Figure 4) (Mattiazzi et al., 2022; Rawlinson et al., 2021; Verhoeven et al., 2021). This multiteam systems thinking is especially important given the breadth of new treatment regimens, the fact that many people diagnosed with cancer are managing other chronic conditions, and because care often occurs in multiple settings and geographic areas (Chollette et al., 2020, 2022).

Weaver stated that multisystem "teaming" can break down when those involved underestimate the time and resources collaboration requires or neglect to view their work as interdependent (Taplin et al., 2015a, 2015b). Therefore, it is important for IPE training to address these potential points of failure, Weaver said, especially as cancer care evolves to include more partnerships with advanced practice providers (APPs), which requires revisiting and clarifying roles, and as new technologies enable more care to occur in patient homes, making patients and their caregivers more active and central team members (Caparso and Friese, 2023; Pickard et al., 2023).

Weaver suggested adopting patient-centered care competencies as critical teamwork priorities. She noted that it is also important to partner with advocacy groups and offer training for caregivers and the public. She said that virtual learning technologies can improve IPE delivery and implementation. Finally, she emphasized that research is needed to assess the effectiveness of multiteam systems in improving care and quality of life for patients, caregivers, and clinicians (Fraher and Brandt, 2019).

The Cancer and Aging Research Group: An Education and Training Network to Facilitate Multidisciplinary, Multispecialty Expert Care

The Cancer and Aging Research Group (CARG) was formed in 2006 to address gaps in geriatric oncology care, said Heidi Klepin, professor of internal medicine, hematology, and oncology at Wake Forest University. She discussed how it could serve as an exemplar of education and training strategies to build multidisciplinary, multispecialty expert care teams.

The majority of patients with a new cancer diagnosis are older adults,[9] but Klepin said the cancer care delivery system is not set up to provide them with quality care (Bluethmann et al., 2016; IOM, 2013). These patients have complex needs and multiple constraints, but there is a lack of evidence from clinical trials on how they respond to cancer therapies, as well as a lack of geriatric clinicians, training, coordination, advocacy, and dedicated resources (Bertagnolli and Singh, 2021; Williams et al., 2020).

---

[9] See https://seer.cancer.gov/statfacts/html/all.html (accessed January 2, 2024).

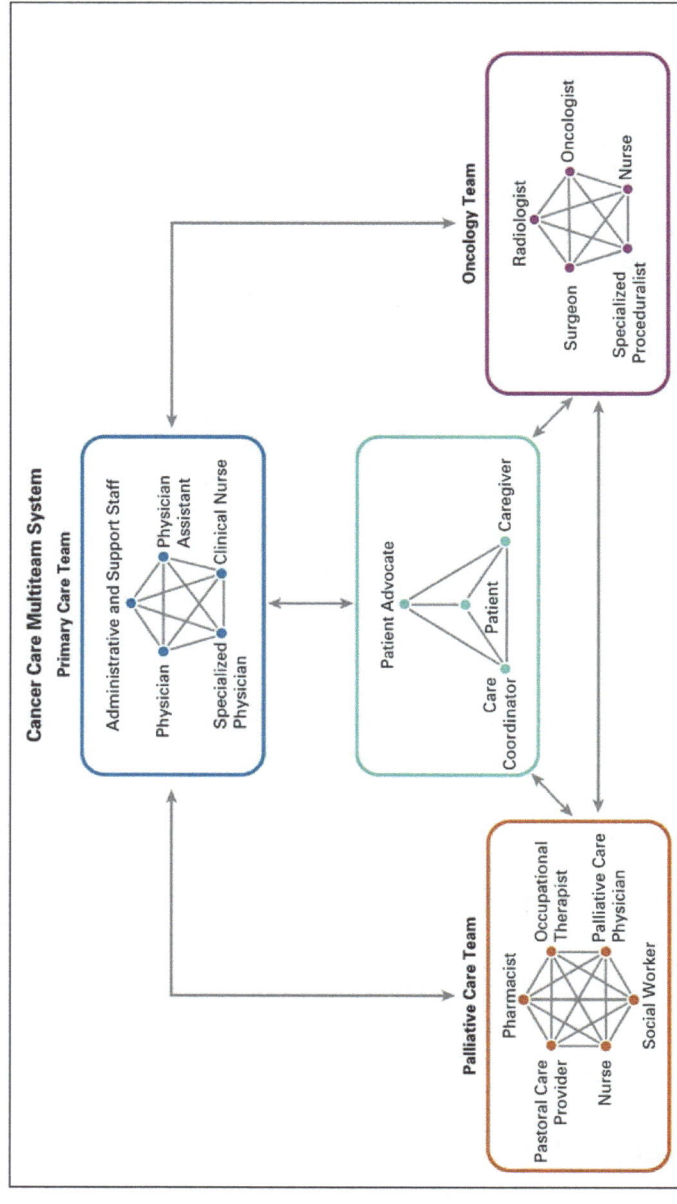

FIGURE 4 Conceptual schematic illustrating an example of a multiteam framework for collaborative cancer care.
SOURCES: Weaver presentation, July 17, 2023. Chollette, V., S. J. Weaver, G. Huang, S. Tsakraklides, and S. P. Tu. 2020. Identifying cancer care team competencies to improve care coordination in multiteam systems: A modified Delphi study. *JCO Oncology Practice* 16(11):e1324–e1331. https://doi.org/10.1200/OP.20.00001.

Klepin explained that the CARG was created to improve the evidence base for treating older adults with cancer and thus improve their quality of care. It is a multidisciplinary, collaborative network whose members conduct research, provide training, and advocate for their patients (Rosko et al., 2021). It has grown into an international organization with more than 600 members and institutional partners, including CHCs and professional organizations, that collaborate to expand the national research infrastructure for interdisciplinary cancer-aging research; conduct research to identify older patients at the highest risk for adverse outcomes from cancer and treatments; develop effective interventions to improve outcomes for these patients and their caregivers; mentor the next generation of aging and cancer researchers; and widely disseminate these findings to improve clinical practice (CARG, 2024).

The CARG has an infrastructure grant with the goal of developing a sustainable national research infrastructure to create and support impactful and innovative projects addressing interdisciplinary research questions at the aging and cancer interface. Priorities include increasing high-impact research, developing effective interventions for older adults and their caregivers, mentoring the next generation of cancer and aging researchers and widely disseminating research findings to inform clinical practice.

Klepin attributed the CARG's success to its clearly defined mission; passionate and engaged participants who created a culture of inclusive collaboration; patient partnerships; creative and noninstitutional thinking; leadership and action opportunities; and an educational pipeline of new colleagues.

Project ECHO: Capacity Building for PCPs in Cancer Survivorship Care

Hilary Ma, associate professor at the University of Texas MD Anderson Cancer Center, described how Project ECHO (Extension of Community Health Outcomes) brings clinicians together to improve survivorship care. The impetus for the project stemmed from challenges faced in coordinating survivorship care across Houston's Harris Health system and its network of clinics, CHCs, and hospitals, which care for a majority-minority population of people who are frequently uninsured, underinsured, or medically underserved. Ma said that most cancer diagnoses originate in primary care clinics; patients are referred to hospitals for cancer treatment and then transitioned back to their PCP because oncologists lack the capacity to see patients indefinitely. As a result, PCPs frequently provide survivorship care, but he said that many feel unprepared to do so.

To solve these challenges and improve survivorship care, Project ECHO's virtual, multidirectional training, educational, and information-sharing platform creates a supportive, mentoring environment that empowers clinicians to improve their knowledge, skills, and patient outcomes. Ma explained that through Project ECHO, cancer center oncologists provide CHC staff and local PCPs with multisession trainings tailored to their needs and focused on issues that are clinically relevant and management and intervention oriented. These sessions cover multiple cancer types and facets of survivorship, such as long-term effects, late effects, physical function, and psychosocial issues. The program has been a success, and subjects report an improved understanding of survivorship issues. Ma suggested that trainings in the ECHO model can be fine-tuned, widely distributed, and scaled up to improve care at safety net health care systems across the country and also applied to different settings and medical specialties.

ENGAGE: Person-Centered Coordinated Care at the Intersection of Cancer and Mental Health

Irwin described Massachusetts General Hospital Cancer Center's ENGAGE program, a diverse, person- and caregiver-centered, strengths-based, multidisciplinary collaborative to facilitate coordinated mental health care for patients with cancer and cancer survivors.[10]

Irwin described the program as grounded in social justice and human rights frameworks and designed to proactively identify patients with specialized mental health needs; address potential barriers to care; create and sustain communities of practice beyond the cancer center and mental health systems; and engage a diverse care team in regular, systematic case reviews to employ evidence-based interventions for cancer and mental illness and reduce cancer care disruptions (Irwin et al., 2017).

ENGAGE operates in a similar way to virtual tumor boards, which are multidisciplinary teams that meet virtually to discuss new or complex cases, decide on a treatment plan, and share best practices (Berardi et al., 2020). However, Irwin clarified that ENGAGE serves as more of a virtual equity board—a coalition of community mental health agencies and cancer centers (that previously did not communicate, despite often treating the same patients) that includes all relevant specialists, draws on community strengths and resources, and facilitates co-learning. She explained that the approach has helped to build a flexible community of practice with the capacity to increase access to psycho-oncology services, educate patients, and overcome care barriers (Irwin et al., 2022).

---

[10] See https://engageinitiative.org/media/ (accessed January 2, 2024).

Supporting Training to Prioritize Access to Care

Many speakers underscored the relationship between the priority placed on improving access to care and the willingness of health systems and clinicians to invest time and resources in education and training programs to facilitate multidisciplinary, multispecialty care. Klepin stated that progress will remain incremental until expanding care access becomes a true priority, backed by financial incentives and institutional support.

Irwin said that a call to action is needed to recognize care inequities as a human rights issue and spur investment in building dedicated programs to address it. Ma agreed, noting that many programs began with one person, "a spark," who was able to move past the systemic barriers endemic to health care and create change. He also added that systemic pressures can create disincentives to participate in changemaking efforts. For example, PCPs may want to participate in training to improve survivorship care but recognize that an hour spent on that would come at the cost of seeing patients, which has financial implications for the practice. Heflin stressed that physicians can support a shared vision of improving survivorship care by advocating for more scheduling flexibility and accommodations.

Heflin noted that most of today's clinicians were trained in one specific discipline and likely have one professional identity, which constrains their ability to work across specialties and disciplines. More multidisciplinary training that blurs the lines between professions, for both active clinicians and trainees, could create the "change agents" needed to build more collaborative care approaches in the future. Gupta agreed and suggested that future physicians also need to be trained as patient advocates: "It is going to be [up to] those doctors who are in training now to change the system."

Ma and Darien emphasized that an expanded, coordinated, collaborative effort and shared framework are needed to address care disparities at a national scale.

HEALTH SYSTEM OPPORTUNITIES

Many speakers emphasized that values, investments, and incentives within health systems can significantly influence the capability to form and sustain functioning multidisciplinary, multispecialty care teams They discussed opportunities to focus attention on the need to improve cancer survivorship care in general and optimize the effectiveness and efficiency of delivering this essential care at the level of health care systems in particular.

The Impetus and Challenge of System-Level Interventions to Support Survivorship

Tevaarwerk and David Dougherty, deputy director of clinical services at the Abramson Cancer Center at the University of Pennsylvania, discussed challenges and opportunities for health systems to deliver multidisciplinary, multispecialty cancer care to the right patient, at the right time, and the right location—and to do so at scale—in the context of a continually evolving cancer care landscape.

The practice of oncology has become more complex as biological discoveries of the past 2 decades have been translated into cancer treatments that require increasingly specialized and multidisciplinary knowledge to administer safely and effectively. Financing for oncology practice is critical to health systems and hospitals, and cancer is a major focus of clinical research, but Dougherty said existing payment models are inadequate to support survivorship care, despite its critical role in patient outcomes. To overcome financial barriers, maximize value, and better serve patients, he suggested that financial analyses are needed to demonstrate revenue gains from expanded survivorship care through an overall value and opportunity cost lens.

Farah Brasfield, regional chief of hematology-oncology at Kaiser Permanente, pointed out that although scientific discoveries, technologies, and new therapies are emerging rapidly, the oncology workforce is shrinking.[11] These two factors make it challenging to deliver the most up-to-date, expert-level care to the nation's growing, and aging, population with cancer. Tevaarwerk highlighted opportunities for health systems to establish system-level accessible and supportive structures and processes through efforts focused on quality integration, service site optimization, expanded advanced care access, and clinical disease teams, and by more effectively leveraging data. At Penn Medicine, for example, multiple structures provide patients at every site in the health system with patient-centered multidisciplinary, multispecialty care pathways to foster cancer survivorship. Tevaarwerk and Dougherty described how Penn Medicine also incentivizes innovation and encourages clinicians to collaborate on system-wide efforts, such as operations, research, strategy, and business development.

Alfano suggested that health care systems also need to hire clinician-leaders to oversee care from diagnosis to survivorship, provide more clinical training, and develop more collaborative technology tools. Health insurers also need to enhance reimbursements to cover navigation and patient self-management, she added. Finally, she said that aligned incentives and metrics for improved clinician and patient experience are critical to support quality survivorship care (see Figure 5) (Alfano et al., 2019, 2022).

---

[11] See https://old-prod.asco.org/sites/new-www.asco.org/files/content-files/news-initiatives/documents/2023-workforce-brief.pdf (accessed January 2, 2024).

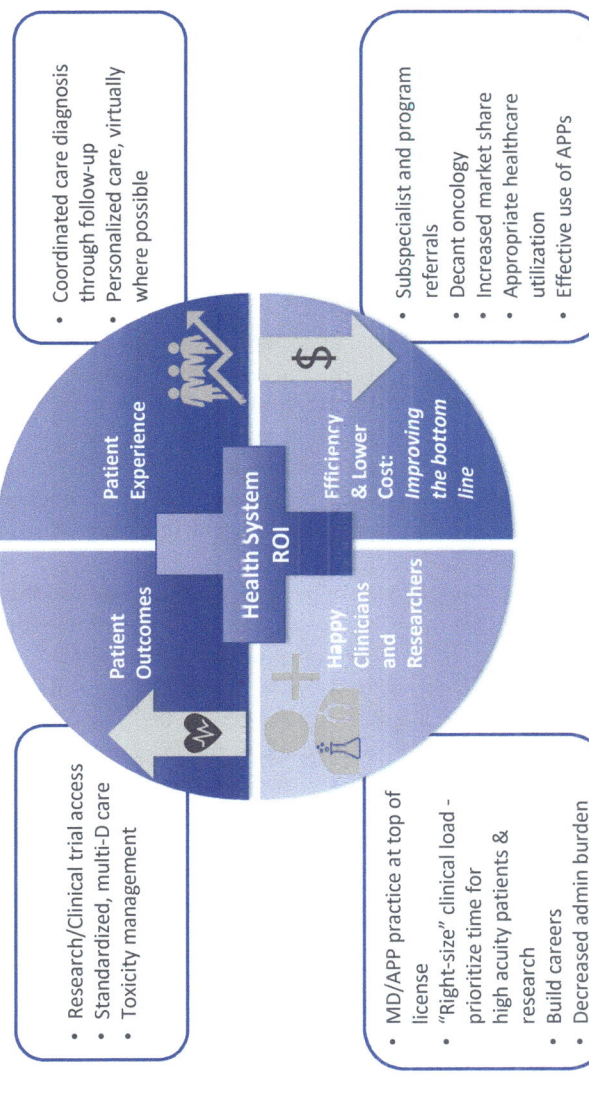

FIGURE 5 Conceptual diagram highlighting areas for which return on investment (ROI) from efforts to improve survivorship care can be assessed across the health system.

NOTE: APP = advanced practice provider; MD = doctor of medicine; Mulit-d = multidisciplinary; ROI = return on investment.

SOURCES: Alfano presentation, July 17, 2023. Alfano, C. M., K. Oeffinger, T. Sanft, and B. Tortorella. 2022. Engaging team medicine in patient care: Redefining cancer survivorship from diagn. osis. *American Society of Clinical Oncology Educational Book* 42:1–11. https://doi.org/10.1200/EDBK_349391.

Integration of Health Systems for Better Cancer Survivorship Care

Brasfield highlighted Kaiser Permanente's new system for care coordination, which is "technology supported, patient centered, and genomics guided." The system encompasses prevention and screening, diagnosis and treatment, and survivorship and surveillance for three population categories: the general population, those at high risk for cancer due to heritable mutations, and those with a history of cancer. The system is designed to coordinate across disciplines and specialties to support personalized, comprehensive, and proactive care pathways. It can interface with EHRs, identify potential adverse effects, suggest treatment and testing pathways, offer nationwide expert case reviews, and integrate cancer clinical trials data and published literature. In addition, she said Kaiser Permanente's digital self-care, telehealth, and in-person wellness programs for survivors deliver integrated, seamless care to support quality of life at every age.

Brasfield stressed that the health care sector needs more innovative approaches like this care coordination system and enhanced payment models for telehealth, greater investment in integrated health care technology, more workforce training in oncology and cancer survivorship, long-term post-treatment studies, and strategies to retain oncologists. She also suggested replacing board exams, which quickly become outdated, with more frequent and structured learning modules that can incorporate emerging research and best practices.

Monica Gramatges, associate professor of pediatrics at the Texas Children's Hospital, described Passport for Care, a clinical decision support tool that translates evidence-based, long-term follow-up guidelines into personalized cancer survivorship care for people with childhood cancer.[12] The tool was created to simplify care plans for the different long-term effects of pediatric treatments, which can vary dramatically depending on the specific cancer. She explained that Passport for Care continually incorporates updated guidelines from the Children's Oncology Group and has improved clinical visits for late effects. Gramatges noted that this tool is poised for wider adoption and can also be adapted to include survivors of adult cancer.

Mary Reid, distinguished professor of oncology at the Roswell Park Comprehensive Cancer Center, described its centralized survivorship program,[13] which was founded on the idea that "survivorship belongs in a cancer center, [but] it doesn't belong in oncology." Now in its 8th year, the program integrates a staff of fully engaged physicians, dieticians, epidemiologists, PTs, social workers, and other specialties to see patients in remote areas of New

---

[12] See https://www.passportforcare.org/en/ (accessed January 2, 2024).
[13] See https://www.roswellpark.org/survivorship (accessed January 2, 2024).

York State. It also recently expanded screening and survivorship services into areas with few community health resources. When they learned that community PCPs lacked time to keep up with the latest research findings, for example, Roswell Park staff shared their knowledge to ensure that CHC patients could receive quality follow-up or survivorship care closer to home, improving patient adherence and quality of life. Reid pointed out that the program's financial strategy captures every cost, ensures that prevention is a sustainable business model, and eases the caseload for cancer centers so that they can focus on caring for patients in active cancer treatment.

Leveraging Data and Technology

Several speakers noted that one way to ensure quality care delivery is to fundamentally change how health systems create, capture, and leverage data for effective population health maintenance and successful patient outcomes. Alfano observed that a risk-and-need stratified model of survivorship care will better meet patient needs and improve clinical efficiency (NHS, 2013), but also noted that implementing such a model at Northwell Health has been challenging because of a lack of structured EHR data. To overcome this barrier, she suggested a collaborative effort to push EHR companies to better incorporate structured data and remote, electronic PRO (ePRO) data that can flag patients in distress, a practice that may require reimbursement changes.

Tevaarwerk described many current systems as "high touch," in which multiple clinicians, patients, and their caregivers manually define, carry out, and review tasks, requiring effort, knowledge, time, and resources. These high-touch processes not only fail to provide extractable structured EHR data, she explained, but they also exacerbate inequities and increases patient and physician burnout, she said. A "high-tech" system, on the other hand, leverages existing—if imperfect—technologies, such as EHRs, to decrease resource-intensive tasks, reduce inequities, and better support clinicians and survivors (Cykert et al., 2020; Tevaarwerk et al., 2018). To implement a high-tech system, Tevaarwerk stressed that EHRs need to move away from manually inputted free text, which usually cannot be integrated into patient portals or care pathways (Cracchiolo et al., 2023; Emamekhoo et al., 2022; Stetson et al., 2022). By contrast, structured and standardized EHR data can be more quickly and easily shared, searched, extracted, and analyzed to improve care delivery (Hassett et al., 2022; Häyrinen and Saranto, 2005; Osterman et al., 2020).

Health systems face substantial challenges in achieving the type of structured data systems that are needed, Tevaarwerk explained. Key challenges include determining who should create these systems, how the use of AI can be optimized, ways to effectively collaborate with EHR vendors, and how to effectively implement new data practices, including gaining necessary approvals and appropriately training staff. Tevaarwerk added that structured data input needs to be prioritized as paid work and should be incorporated into consensus guidelines. Moreover, she stressed that data input should be tracked, and these data should be leveraged as much as possible. She said that implementing and sustaining data-based strategies requires providing sufficient system support, IT services, and financial resources (Gabriel et al., 2023).

Brasfield pointed out that oncology practices do not have sufficient staff to take on additional data entry tasks, which are extremely time intensive. Gramatges agreed, noting that Passport for Care requires an initial data entry procedure that some clinicians have found to be a barrier. In addition, there are challenges with data interoperability across institutions.

Tevaarwerk and Dougherty agreed that the lack of novel EHR tools to capture more structured, translatable data results in lost opportunities. Tevaarwerk noted that relying on AI tools can be useful, but they can also increase disparities if they are developed without data from historically marginalized populations: "One of the things that makes me very nervous about AI is that it is only as good as the data it is fed." Darien agreed and pointed out that the AI training data available today are not representative of the general population and cannot capture critically important nuances. Marlyn Allicock, assistant professor at the University of Texas, Dallas, said that AI tools can fail to capture more subjective measures, such as mental health symptoms, that are harder for clinicians to translate into data.

Brasfield stressed the need for new data tools to be simple, automated, and seamless. Tevaarwerk agreed, adding that they should also be interoperable, so that patient registries, EHRs, and other systems can share information. Dougherty suggested that these tools need to utilize structured data elements to better capture and share information across systems. Shulman added that changes to reimbursements from CMS and private insurance plans can incentivize the use of structured data. For example, Penn Medicine uses a "smart form" that turns input into structured, extractable data, which he said could be emulated on a national scale with a strong advocacy campaign. "If all we're going to do is tweak the system and add something on top of it, it won't work," he stated. "We need to change the basic rules of the system."

Learning from Other Fields of Medicine

The cancer care community could learn from the standards of care for other diseases, Alfano suggested. For example, diabetes and asthma care place more emphasis on self-management and have standardized metrics and insurance reimbursements. Nekhlyudov pointed out that each type of cancer is more like its own separate, distinct disease, which limits the ability to learn from other disease categories.

Brasfield suggested that oncologists can also learn from the workflows of other clinical settings. PCPs, for example, have experience with a high volume of patients and complex cases. Tevaarwerk noted that the tools her organization created were inspired by tools used in other care settings. Alfano added that successful models for survivorship care in cancer could also be expanded into other disciplines.

System-Level Efforts to Reduce Health Disparities

Multilevel efforts that include patients, clinicians, health care systems, and policies can play an essential role in reducing health disparities across the cancer continuum, observed Allicock. She suggested that clinicians need to better incorporate the patient perspectives into survivorship care programs, increase patient engagement and self-management, and support patients as they navigate the entire cancer care continuum. She added that health care systems should partner with CHCs to address SDOH that contribute to racial disparities in health outcomes by creating access and support for entities that have built trust with their communities. Reid agreed, saying "It's not a matter of them trusting us, it's that we have to engage the people they trust." Allicock noted that it would be helpful to optimize virtual care services—including clinician training and infrastructure support—to address the frequently changing circumstances and unique health challenges of adolescent and young adult cancer survivors (Shay et al., 2022).

Brasfield suggested that establishing mobile clinics and volunteer programs in medically underserved communities could help to better reach those who have less access to technology or prefer in-home visits. Alfano stated that her system hires community members who speak the languages of the community, which creates "cancer cultural ambassadors" who can help with complex conversations. Reid and Gramatges suggested that survivorship programs should find ways to partner more effectively with PCPs, who are often the only local resource for cancer survivors and help them identify the appropriate survivorship guidelines or care pathways. "It's really important that we utilize and strengthen that relationship with them," Reid stated.

Winn suggested that health care systems should hire community members to perform structured data entry, which would create new jobs, elevate communities, and provide more visibility for "data deserts." These "data extenders" would be analogous to the extension mission of land-grant universities, he said.

Darien noted that patients are still being left out of the conversation. It will take intentional, collaborative discussions to ensure that clinicians understand each patient as well as the overall system to provide the best care and support needed changes.

POLICY, PAYMENT, AND ADVOCACY OPPORTUNITIES

Many of the challenges to achieving multidisciplinary, multispecialty survivorship care at the system level stem from issues related to policy and payment structures, noted many speakers. In addition, many speakers highlighted structural barriers confronting patients with cancer in the United States, and how they influence the function of health systems. Many speakers also identified potential opportunities to advocate for transformative changes that could significantly enhance survivorship care.

The Human Toll of Policy and Payment Challenges

Shortcomings in health care policy and payment structures in the United States result in significant burdens on patients and their families, said Stacie Dusetzina, professor of health policy at the Vanderbilt University School of Medicine. She said that a substantial portion of the U.S. population cannot afford basic health care, much less the multidisciplinary, multispecialty care that cancer survivors need.

The much higher spending on cancer care in the United States compared with most developed nations does not translate into a lower cancer mortality rate, noted Robin Yabroff, scientific vice president of health services research at the American Cancer Society (Chow et al., 2022). Multiple speakers discussed contributors to these poor outcomes. A key issue is the racial and socioeconomic disparities in access to cancer prevention, screening, and treatment, which are correlated with mortality rates (see Figure 6) (Islami et al., 2022; Singh and Jemal, 2017). Yabroff noted that these disparities exist across the entire care continuum but are often exacerbated for those with long-term adverse effects from cancer treatment, who need well-coordinated specialty care. Such adverse effects can limit these survivors' ability to work, risking the loss of household income and employer-sponsored health insurance for themselves and their families. Remaining employed, however, can make it difficult to schedule clinic appointments and adhere to complex treatment plans.

In addition to demographic disparities, Yabroff explained that gaps in health insurance coverage (see Figure 7) affect cancer mortality. People with more serious diagnoses who have private insurance often fare better than people without insurance, even those with less advanced cancer (Zhao et al., 2022). People without insurance are also more likely to experience serious financial hardships due to medical care. However, all cancer survivors, even those with health insurance, report financial hardships and treatment barriers, such as coverage gaps and disruptions, high deductibles, fear of job loss, and transportation issues (Han et al., 2020; MacKinnon et al., 2023; Shankaran et al., 2022; Yabroff et al., 2018; Zheng et al., 2020). In short, health insurance

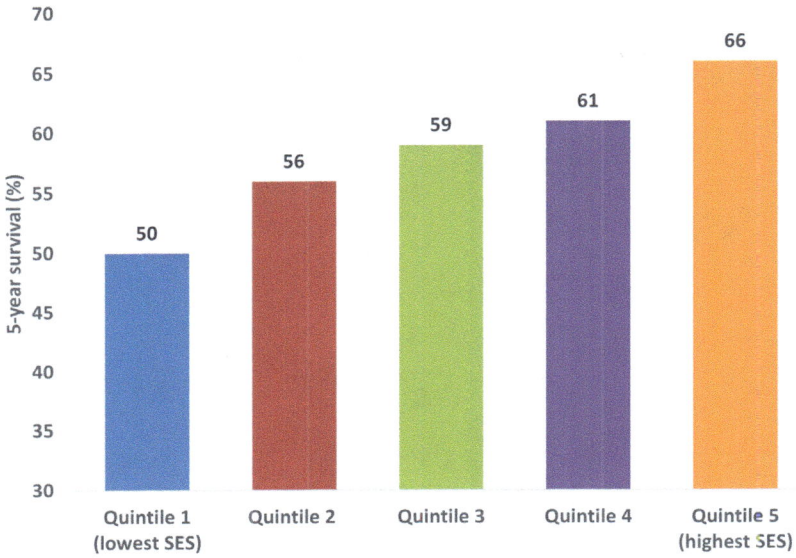

FIGURE 6 Five-year survival following cancer diagnosis in the United States by socioeconomic status quintile.
NOTE: SES = socioeconomic status.
SOURCES: Yabroff presentation, July 18, 2023; Singh and Jemal, 2017. (Copyright © 2017 Gopal K. Singh and Ahmedin Jemal, distributed under the Creative Commons Attribution License).

coverage is no guarantee that an average person will be able to access or afford the health care they need, said Yabroff.

Closing Gaps in Insurance Coverage for Survivorship Care

Although the overall number of uninsured people in the Unites States has declined since the implementation of the Affordable Care Act (ACA), Dusetzina noted that programs still need significant improvements to support better access to health care in general and cancer survivorship care in particular. First, she argued that Medicaid should be expanded in all states to close the coverage gap of nearly 2 million people. Some populations in need find it virtually impossible to qualify for Medicaid in states without Medicaid expansion, and they cannot afford private insurance even with federal subsidies. In addition, she stressed that it is important to eliminate administrative barriers

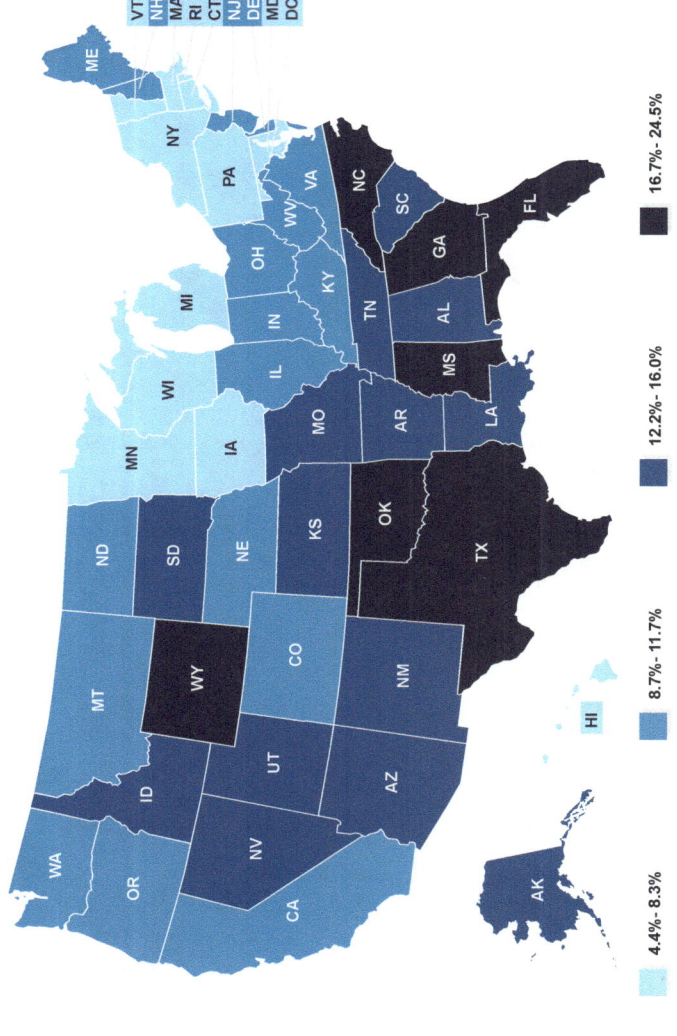

FIGURE 7 Percentage of adults aged 19–64 years without health insurance coverage by state in 2019.
SOURCES: Yabroff presentation, July 18, 2023. Uninsured rates for the nonelderly by age (KFF, 2023). https://www.kff.org/uninsured/state-indicator/nonelderly-uninsured-rate-by-age/?activeTab= map&currentTimeframe=2&selectedDistributions=adults-19-64&sortModel=%7B%22colId%22:%22Location%22,%22sort%22:%22asc%22%7D (accessed April 3, 2024); CC BY-NC-ND 4.0.

that unjustly disenroll eligible people from Medicaid. Sara Rosenbaum, professor emerita of health law and policy at George Washington University also suggested that Medicaid coverage be expanded to include the full standard of care for patients with cancer.

Looking specifically at the Medicare program, Dusetzina said that reforms are needed to address significant coverage gaps, burdensome administrative tasks, high costs, and confusing eligibility rules. She also argued that Medicare needs an out-of-pocket spending cap for patients; although Medigap[14] was created to reduce coverage gaps, it has confusing eligibility rules and unexpectedly high premiums and treatment costs. Medicare Advantage,[15] which is provided by private plans, offers more coverage and benefits, but enrollees report fewer in-network clinicians and more out-of-network costs and may find it difficult to switch back to traditional Medicare if they are dissatisfied.

The ACA created a health insurance marketplace where those who are not eligible for Medicare, Medicaid, or employer-sponsored insurance can buy their own plan and will not be denied coverage because of prior cancer diagnoses or other pre-existing conditions. These plans have out-of-pocket spending caps, but these caps are still high, and the overall cost for premiums is out of reach for many, Dusetzina said. Rosenbaum suggested that Congress authorize enhanced subsidies to people excluded from Medicaid so they can obtain insurance through the marketplace. Also, she said that all marketplace plans should be reviewed to ensure adequate provider team care coverage. For example, she said that team care would be more widely adopted if reimbursements were increased and telehealth and supportive services could improve access in rural and underserved communities.

Survivorship care also raises unique issues, such as complex dental care needs. Jennifer Perkins, assistant dean of education at the University of California, San Francisco, noted that cancer survivors often have complex dentistry needs and require high-quality, timely care tailored to their specific disease and treatment effects, but this level of care is very difficult to obtain, even when it should technically be covered by private insurance, Medicare, or Medicaid. Very few dental clinics accept Medicaid because the reimbursements are very low, and there are no dental codes associated with cancer care. In addition, traditional Medicare excludes dental services. The dental workforce also lacks training in caring for patients with cancer.

To address these gaps, Perkins highlighted the need for new reimbursement codes for complex dental care, incentives for rural dentists to accept

---

[14] See https://www.cms.gov/medicare/health-drug-plans/medigap (accessed March 13, 2024).

[15] See https://www.medicare.gov/Pubs/pdf/12026-Understanding-Medicare-Advantage-Plans.pdf (accessed March 13, 2024).

Medicaid, and improved training on Medicaid billing for dental clinics. She also suggested incorporating the unique dental needs of cancer survivors into standard dental curricula. Stout added that West Virginia recently created a working group on cancer rehabilitation and oral health to address some of the issues Perkins identified.

Ideas and Efforts to Improve Payment and Service Delivery Models

Yabroff pointed out that smarter, more efficient health care spending is needed to address the health and financial issues all patients face—whether insured or uninsured. Several approaches have been employed to address payment and policy barriers and improve cancer care and survivorship care delivery.

Hillary Cavanagh, director of ambulatory payment models at the CMS Innovation Center, described the Center's testing of new payment and service delivery models to improve care and reduce costs. The CMS Oncology Care Model, for example, created significant care improvements, including a reduction in higher-risk cancers, but incurred a net financial loss. A newer iteration, the Enhancing Oncology Model (EOM), is not a typical fee-for-service model. Rather, participants are financially responsible for the total care costs over 6 months, with performance-based reimbursements. The EOM focuses on fewer cancer types; increases payments for more complex care; emphasizes patient-centered care and enhanced services, such as navigation and ePROs; and employs home health registered nurses to screen for and address health disparities or barriers. Its goals—to better support patients with cancer and improve care—also align with the goals of the Cancer Moonshot Initiative,[16] Cavanagh noted.

Cavanagh observed that the EOM can help to avoid adverse patient outcomes by focusing on financial accountability. Its performance-based payments are tied to specific quality measures that align with patient outcomes, which are tracked via real-time patient monitoring systems. The EOM has broader goals of addressing health disparities and enabling more patient-centric care through enhanced services, such as patient navigation, care planning, clinical guideline compliance, and ePROs. EOM participants are also required to have an evidence-based health equity plan to address care disparities.

Shulman described efforts by the Commission on Cancer (CoC),[17] which uses defined standards to accredit about 1,500 cancer programs that together serve nearly 70 percent of the U.S. population newly diagnosed with cancer.

---

[16] See https://www.whitehouse.gov/cancermoonshot/ (accessed March 26, 2024).

[17] See https://www.facs.org/quality-programs/cancer-programs/commission-on-cancer/ (accessed January 3, 2024).

In 2012, the CoC introduced a new standard requiring programs to provide survivorship care plans, but nearly every program struggled to meet this standard. Several groups, such as the CoC, NCI, and ASCO, collaborated to revise the standard to focus on creating structured survivorship programs, with designated leaders and improvement targets. Survivorship care is now more of a priority at cancer centers, but Shulman cautioned that it is too early to tell how much progress has been made.

Emily Tonorezos, director of the Office of Cancer Survivorship at NCI, discussed work that the office is doing to support survivorship care. She said that these efforts are driven by a focus on prioritizing and funding research that benefits all patients with cancer, as well as their caregivers; does not worsen care disparities or inequities; and centers the patient experience. She pointed out that this research is especially important because many patients find that a cancer diagnosis worsens their financial circumstances and thus adds barriers to accessing multidisciplinary, multispecialty care. Yabroff and Shulman suggested that NCI could also develop high-quality, multidisciplinary survivorship care models to use in cancer center evaluation and accreditation.

Policy Options to Facilitate Care Coordination and Navigation

Shelley Fuld Nasso, the chief executive officer of the National Coalition for Cancer Survivorship noted that patients face many challenges accessing care—whether they have insurance or not. Moreover, patients incur a significant financial and mental burden in coordinating their own care, which can exacerbate inequities. To reduce these burdens, she stressed the importance of care planning, starting at the time of diagnosis. She added that the EOM covers care planning, but a new, cancer-specific billing code[18] is necessary for coordinated patient navigation through traditional Medicare. Fuld Nasso also advocated for passage of the Comprehensive Cancer Survivorship Act,[19] which would provide coverage for cancer care planning and navigation and support clinician training for survivorship care.

Jennifer Malin, senior vice president and chief medical officer at Optum Health Solutions, called for the creation of a new category of specialists to focus on the diverse, complex, and often expensive issues of cancer survivors (and other complex diseases) and to coordinate multidisciplinary, multispecialty care to prevent or mitigate long-term adverse effects. These "thrivists" would have the expertise to optimally manage coordinated care and treatment

---

[18] See https://www.cms.gov/files/document/mln9201074-health-equity-services-2024-physician-fee-schedule-final-rule.pdf-0 (accessed April 1, 2024).

[19] See https://canceradvocacy.org/policy/comprehensive-cancer-survivorship-act-ccsa/ (accessed March 26, 2024).

effects at scale, relieving patients of this burden. This position would also create new opportunities to conduct clinical research, reform payment models, and advocate for innovations in policy, payment, research, and care delivery.

In Malin's view, creating a new survivorship specialty could create a focal point for new services, voices, and experiences, similar to the growth of palliative care, and reduce survivors' invisible suffering through the aid of a designated "quarterback." Tonorezos suggested that CARG would be a good model for education and training to build teams. Choi and Fuld Nasso added that PCPs could be well suited for this role, although there is a projected PCP shortage (HRSA, 2024). Jacobs added that 2 decades of research demonstrates that oncology APPs are in a good position to coordinate cancer survivorship care. With the right support and training, she suggested that APPs could address many of the challenges discussed at this workshop.

Alternative Payment Models

"How do we think about making our healthcare dollars go farther [. . .] so that we don't just have more spending, but we have more efficient spending?" Dusetzina asked. She suggested focusing more effort on drug price negotiations and noted that eliminating reimbursements for high-cost, low-value drugs could free up resources for survivorship care. Aligning reimbursements with the value of a service or therapy—a common practice in other countries—would also reward companies that create beneficial therapies and improve patient outcomes, she posited.

Perkins agreed that value-based payment models enable more flexibility and service offerings, but, given that even patients with private insurance face high costs, she said that changes to insurance policies that define patient cost sharing are needed to minimize financial barriers. She also noted that more clarity on the potential benefits and risks of treatments, both short and long term, would help patients and caregivers make informed health and financial decisions. Yabroff suggested enabling Medicare to use cost effectiveness data analyses in coverage decisions. Fuld Nasso noted that data demonstrating the cost effectiveness of new interventions could facilitate implementation and adoption and that clinical trials should collect data on the financial and emotional costs for patients and caregivers.

Fuld Nasso also suggested that people living with metastatic cancers can benefit from and should be included in survivorship programs. Christopher Friese, the Elizabeth Tone Hosmer professor of nursing at the University of Michigan, expressed optimism that various care models discussed at the workshop could inspire reimbursement policy changes to cover new services and expand cancer care team capabilities while controlling costs but noted that the support of institutions and health systems will also be essential for success.

The Power of Perceptions of Value on Patient-, Clinician-, and System-Level Decisions

Stout expressed frustration that clinicians are asked to work more efficiently and justify their costs, whereas new, expensive therapies are routinely reimbursed, even when they provide little survival benefit. She said support services are just as critical to patients surviving and thriving and deserve more payment equity, yet she sees "a huge disparity in how we're choosing to cut the pie."

Carlson suggested the "cost of care" should be reframed as a "life cycle of care" to encompass both immediate costs and longer-term costs—as well as the longer-term savings that survivorship care can bring. Darien emphasized that clinical care costs should also incorporate contributions of CHC staff, who often work more closely with community members than hospital-based navigators and can be well positioned to fill gaps in survivorship care.

Shulman pointed out that cancer centers rely on the revenue from expensive treatments, which would not change even with new payment models. Dusetzina said that bundled payments provide better value and more tailored care than fee-for-service models. Centers that provide efficient, effective care would perform better financially, she noted. Yabroff cautioned that new payment models could unintentionally exacerbate inequities, because centers, driven by financial pressures, might turn away patients with complex needs. Darien noted that the Patient-Centered Outcomes Research Institute was recently authorized to study patients' economic burdens to improve equity. "It is not just being an accountant but also being an economist, to really look at what the burdens are overall, not just the burdens of cost of health care," Darien said.

Facilitating Effective Team-Based Care

Brasfield said that most cancer centers do not use team-based, integrated care approaches, and as a result, the oncology workforce is overly burdened by treatments and procedures that are easily reimbursed, in addition to the more complex, less reimbursable quality-of-life areas of care. To adequately recognize the time clinicians spend on survivorship care, Choi suggested using time-based billing that also accounts for tasks outside the day of service, such as care coordination efforts between clinical visits.

Shulman acknowledged that structural issues keep many specialists siloed, and workforce shortages can determine each individual clinician's bandwidth and willingness to work collaboratively. To make meaningful progress, he suggested that institutions should prioritize resources and nonhierarchical team-based strategies where the need is highest. He also noted that the CoC's standard for survivorship care requires team-based care to help oncology clinicians see beyond the acute treatment phase and improve the overall patient experience. Carlson and Shulman agreed that promoting teamwork is also a cultural issue. "Without the right culture," Carlson said, "a team will never appropriately function."

Tonorezos noted that tumor boards are an effective model for collaboration and could incorporate survivorship care into their goals. Cavanagh said that daily or weekly team huddles may improve patient navigation and better meet patients' complex medical and psychosocial needs. Perkins said that cancer centers that co-locate care improve the patient experience, especially those with patient navigators, whose ability to take on clinicians' "invisible workload" make the biggest difference. Although adding staff is a large upfront investment, Perkins emphasized that it has been shown to result in more care and better patient outcomes (Natale-Pereira et al., 2011).

The Quest for Equity

Tonorezos and Yabroff underscored that the inequities experienced in the United States are myriad, unjust, and expensive. Given the dearth of safety net programs, Yabroff said that it is important to recognize that health care policies intersect with other issues, such as employment status and sick leave benefits, that do not necessarily fit within health care but are nonetheless important for overall health.

Winn observed that health care in the United States is not only dysfunctional but disconnected. The pieces—CHCs, academic research centers, and comprehensive cancer centers—are not structurally connected. Instead of fighting over resources, he urged the health community to focus on connecting the support and research structures to drive improvements.

Heflin posited that equitable care will not occur as a by-product of other models; achieving it will require a dedicated equity model. He said one example is the Program of All-Inclusive Care for the Elderly,[20] which provides team-based care at community centers that includes transportation, nutrition, therapy, recreation, and caregiver support. Darien noted that centering patients' values and economic burdens is fundamental to delivering equitable multispeciality, multidisciplinary care.

CLOSING DISCUSSION

Brasfield and Shulman said that implementing the improvements suggested over the course of the workshop would require partnerships between

---

[20] See https://www.medicaid.gov/medicaid/long-term-services-supports/program-all-inclusive-care-elderly/index.html (accessed January 5, 2024).

oncology and information technology specialists, noting that medicine has been slow to incorporate the technology and data collection needed to drive the development of usable patient and clinician platforms that support efficient care and improve patient outcomes.

Technology could also be used to measure patients' time burdens incurred by follow-up care, Dusetzina suggested. Shulman shared that research has demonstrated that this "staggering" time burden for patients—from commuting to and from appointments to sitting in waiting rooms and receiving care—can have important implications for their quality of life, and also their household income for any time away from work, because most care is delivered during the traditional work week (Dood et al., 2018; Yabroff et al., 2021). Darien added that patients also have heavy administrative burdens, and the best way to determine what a patient wants is to ask them, trust them, and empower them to ensure that treatment and care decisions truly align with their life goals.

Weaver noted that NCI's Healthcare Delivery Research Program is building the evidence base for team care; she highlighted opportunities for funding and encouraged experts in oncology care to participate in the research peer review process. In addition, she described an NCI conference focused on measurement of teaming and team-based care in cancer care delivery.[21] Yabroff emphasized that increased coordinated team care utilization could lead to fewer emergency department visits and hospital stays, reducing overall costs and improving patient and caregiver outcomes.

Clinicians also need clear and accessible guidelines to implement improved survivorship care, Klepin said. She shared that ASCO's newest evidence-based survivorship guidelines require clinicians to conduct multidimensional, holistic, geriatric assessments (which are adaptable for younger patients) during treatment to trigger needed interventions, minimize adverse and late effects, and improve patient satisfaction. Challenges in paying for or prioritizing this practice, especially in underresourced areas, can be overcome through roadmaps that directly connect patients and services, Klepin suggested. Nekhlyudov agreed, noting that a tailored assessment for survivorship rehabilitation would be enormously helpful.

Stout highlighted the need to share more details on survivorship care models, including core standards, internal goalposts, and acceptable variations that differentiate "standardized care" from the ability to treat a patient's unique needs. Carlson commented that these should be based on evidence from multiple large clinical trials with very high concordance levels and that "value" has different meanings, such as care efficacy, relationships, cost effectiveness, or care quality, so it is important to specify which definition is being used.

---

[21] See https://healthcaredelivery.cancer.gov/media/measures-and-methods.html (accessed April 3, 2024).

Roy Jensen, vice chancellor and director of the University of Kansas Cancer Center, observed that many speakers lamented the lack of a coordinated U.S. health care system. As a result, survivorship care varies widely, patient-facing clinicians lack time and resources to coordinate care, and very little structural support or compensation exists for team-based care. Klepin reiterated that quality survivorship care requires a consistent care leader, starting at diagnosis.

Thomson suggested employing decision and implementation scientists and engaging with the Cancer Prevention and Control Research Network[22] to facilitate adoption of these changes. Irwin agreed, adding that incorporating person-centered and flexible health equity practices should be a priority. "Everybody doesn't need everything, but some populations clearly need different things," she stated. Peterson suggested creating a road map for researchers, clinicians, health economists, and others in the cancer care community to collaboratively work toward improving multidisciplinary, multispecialty care for cancer survivors and their families.

REFERENCES

ACS (American Cancer Society). 2019. *Cancer Treatment & Survivorship Facts & Figures 2019-2021.* https://www.cancer.org/content/dam/cancer-org/research/cancer-facts-and-statistics/cancer-treatment-and-survivorship-facts-and-figures/cancer-treatment-and-survivorship-facts-and-figures-2019-2021.pdf (accessed November 27, 2023).

ACS. 2023. *Cancer Facts and Figures.* https://www.cancer.org/content/dam/cancer-org/research/cancer-facts-and-statistics/annual-cancer-facts-and-figures/2023/2023-cancer-facts-and-figures.pdf (accessed August 11, 2023).

Adusumalli, S., G. P. Kanter, D. S. Small, D. A. Asch, K. G. Volpp, S. H. Park, Y. Gitelman, D. Do, D. Leri, C. Rhodes, C. VanZandbergen, J. T. Howell, M. Epps, A. M. Cavella, M. Wenger, T. O. Harrington, K. Clark, J. E. Westover, C. K. Snider, and M. S. Patel. 2023. Effect of nudges to clinicians, patients, or both to increase statin prescribing: A cluster randomized clinical trial. *JAMA Cardiology* 8(1):23–30.

Alfano, C. M., D. K. Mayer, S. Bhatia, J. Maher, J. M. Scott, L. Nekhlyudov, J. K. Merrill, and T. O. Henderson. 2019. Implementing personalized pathways for cancer follow-up care in the United States: Proceedings from an American Cancer Society–American Society of Clinical Oncology summit. *CA: A Cancer Journal for Clinicians* 69(3):234–247.

Alfano, C. M., K. Oeffinger, T. Sanft, and B. Tortorella. 2022. Engaging team medicine in patient care: Redefining cancer survivorship from diagnosis. *American Society of Clinical Oncology Educational Book* 42:1–11.

---

[22] See https://cpcrn.org/ (accessed April 1, 2024).

Alvarez-Cardona, J. A., J. Ray, J. Carver, V. Zaha, R. Cheng, E. Yang, J. D. Mitchell, K. Stockerl-Goldstein, L. Kondapalli, S. Dent, A. Arnold, S. A. Brown, M. Leja, A. Barac, D. J. Lenihan, and J. Herrmann. 2020. Cardio-oncology education and training: JACC Council perspectives. *Journal of the American College of Cardiology* 76(19):2267–2281.

Arends, J., V. Baracos, H. Bertz, F. Bozzetti, P. C. Calder, N. E. P. Deutz, N. Erickson, A. Laviano, M. P. Lisanti, D. N. Lobo, D. C. McMillan, M. Muscaritoli, J. Ockenga, M. Pirlich, F. Strasser, M. de van der Schueren, A. Van Gossum, P. Vaupel, and A. Weimann. 2017. ESPEN expert group recommendations for action against cancer-related malnutrition. *Clinical Nutrition* 36(5):1187–1196.

Armenian, S. H., L. Xu, B. Ky, C. Sun, L. T. Farol, S. K. Pal, P. S. Douglas, S. Bhatia, and C. Chao. 2016. Cardiovascular disease among survivors of adult-onset cancer: A community-based retrospective cohort study. *Journal of Clinical Oncology* 34(10):1122–1130.

ASCO (American Society of Clinical Oncology). 2020. *Key Trends in Tracking Supply of and Demand for Oncologists*. https://old-prod.asco.org/sites/new-www.asco.org/files/content-files/practice-and-guidelines/documents/2020-workforce-information-system.pdf (accessed August 11, 2023).

Azriful, E. Bujawati, Nildawati, R. Ramdan, F. Mallapiang, and S. Suyuti. 2021. Health belief model on women's cancer recovery (a phenomenological study on cancer survivors). *Gaceta Sanitaria* 35(Suppl 1):S9–S11.

Babiker, A., M. El Husseini, A. Al Nemri, A. Al Frayh, N. Al Juryyan, M. O. Faki, A. Assiri, M. Al Saadi, F. Shaikh, and F. Al Zamil. 2014. Health care professional development: Working as a team to improve patient care. *Sudanese Journal of Paediatrics* 14(2):9–16.

Barnes, C. A., N. L. Stout, T. K. Varghese, Jr., C. M. Ulrich, D. R. Couriel, C. J. Lee, C. S. Noren, and P. C. LaStayo. 2020. Clinically integrated physical therapist practice in cancer care: A new comprehensive approach. *Physical Therapy* 100(3):543–553.

Beck, A. J., C. Page, J. Buche, D. Rittman, and M. Gaiser. 2018. *Estimating the distribution of the U.S. psychiatric subspecialist workforce.* Ann Arbor, MI: University of Michigan Behavioral Health Workforce Research Center.

Bell, C. F., X. Lei, A. Haas, R. A. Baylis, H. Gao, L. Luo, S. H. Giordano, M. R. Wehner, K. T. Nead, and N. J. Leeper. 2023. Risk of cancer after diagnosis of cardiovascular disease. *JACC CardioOncology* 5(4):431–440.

Berardi, R., F. Morgese, S. Rinaldi, M. Torniai, G. Mentrasti, L. Scortichini, and R. Giampieri. 2020. Benefits and limitations of a multidisciplinary approach in cancer patient management. *Cancer Management and Research* 12:9363–9374.

Bertagnolli, M. M., and H. Singh. 2021. Treatment of older adults with cancer—Addressing gaps in evidence. *New England Journal of Medicine* 385(12):1062–1065.

Bertero, E., F. Robusto, E. Rulli, A. D'Ettorre, L. Bisceglia, L. Staszewsky, C. Maack, V. Lepore, R. Latini, and P. Ameri. 2022. Cancer incidence and mortality according to pre-existing heart failure in a community-based cohort. *JACC CardioOncology* 4(1):98–109.

Bluethmann, S. M., A. B. Mariotto, and J. H. Rowland. 2016. Anticipating the "silver tsunami": Prevalence trajectories and comorbidity burden among older cancer survivors in the United States. *Cancer Epidemiology, Biomarkers & Prevention* 25(7):1029–1036.

Bogossian, F., K. New, K. George, N. Barr, N. Dodd, A. L. Hamilton, G. Nash, N. Masters, F. Pelly, C. Reid, R. Shakhovskoy, and J. Taylor. 2023. The implementation of interprofessional education: A scoping review. *Advances in Health Science Education* 28(1):243–277.

Bossi, P., P. Delrio, A. Mascheroni, and M. Zanetti. 2021. The spectrum of malnutrition/cachexia/sarcopenia in oncology according to different cancer types and settings: A narrative review. *Nutrients* 13(6).

CARG (Cancer and Aging Research Group). 2024. *Scoreboard.* https://www.mycarg.org/?page_id=148 (accessed March 13, 2024).

Caparso, C., and C. R. Friese. 2023. Technology supports to cancer care teams: Promises and pitfalls. *JCO Oncology Practice* 19(1):13–15.

Chan, R. J., F. Crawford-Williams, M. Crichton, R. Joseph, N. H. Hart, K. Milley, P. Druce, J. Zhang, M. Jefford, K. Lisy, J. Emery, and L. Nekhlyudov. 2023. Effectiveness and implementation of models of cancer survivorship care: An overview of systematic reviews. *Journal of Cancer Survivorship* 17(1):197–221.

Cheville, A. L., T. Moynihan, J. R. Basford, J. A. Nyman, M. L. Tuma, D. A. Macken, T. Therneau, D. Satelel, and K. Kroenke. 2018. The rationale, design, and methods of a randomized, controlled trial to evaluate the effectiveness of collaborative telecare in preserving function among patients with late stage cancer and hematologic conditions. *Contemporary Clinical Trials* 64:254–264.

Cheville, A. L., T. Moynihan, J. Herrin, C. Loprinzi, and K. Kroenke. 2019. Effect of collaborative telerehabilitation on functional impairment and pain among patients with advanced-stage cancer: A randomized clinical trial. *JAMA Oncology* 5(5):644–652.

Chollette, V., S. J. Weaver, G. Huang, S. Tsakraklides, and S. P. Tu. 2020. Identifying cancer care team competencies to improve care coordination in multiteam systems: A modified Delphi study. *JCO Oncology Practice* 16(11):e1324–e1331.

Chollette, V., M. Doose, J. Sanchez, and S. J. Weaver. 2022. Teamwork competencies for interprofessional cancer care in multiteam systems: A narrative synthesis. *Journal of Interprofessional Care* 36(4):617–625.

Chow, R. D., E. H. Bradley, and C. P. Gross. 2022. Comparison of cancer-related spending and mortality rates in the U.S. vs. 21 high-income countries. *JAMA Health Forum* 3(5):e221229.

Cracchiolo, J. R., W. Arafat, A. Atreja, L. Bruckner, H. Emamekhoo, T. Heinrichs, A. C. Raldow, J. Smerage, P. Stetson, J. Sugalski, and A. J. Tevaarwerk. 2023. Getting ready for real-world use of electronic patient-reported outcomes (ePROs) for patients with cancer: A National Comprehensive Cancer Network EPRO Workgroup paper. *Cancer* 129(16):2441–2449.

Cykert, S., E. Eng, M. A. Manning, L. B. Robertson, D. E. Heron, N. S. Jones, J. C. Schaal, A. Lightfoot, H. Zhou, C. Yongue, and Z. Gizlice. 2020. A multi-faceted intervention aimed at Black–White disparities in the treatment of early stage cancers: The ACCURE pragmatic quality improvement trial. *Journal of the National Medical Association* 112(5):468–477.

Deepak, J. A., X. Ng, J. Feliciano, L. Mao, and A. J. Davidoff. 2015. Pulmonologist involvement, stage-specific treatment, and survival in adults with non-small cell lung cancer and chronic obstructive pulmonary disease. *Annals of the American Thoracic Society* 12(5):742–751.

Demissei, B. G., S. Adusumalli, R. A. Hubbard, S. Denduluri, V. Narayan, A. S. Clark, P. Shah, H. Knollman, K. D. Getz, R. Aplenc, J. R. Carver, and B. Ky. 2020. Cardiology involvement in patients with breast cancer treated with trastuzumab. *JACC CardioOncology* 2(2):179–189.

Deshields, T., B. Zebrack, and V. Kennedy. 2013. The state of psychosocial services in cancer care in the United States. *Psycho-Oncology* 22(3):699–703.

Dood, R. L., Y. Zhao, S. D. Armbruster, R. L. Coleman, S. Tworoger, A. K. Sood, and K. A. Baggerly. 2018. Defining survivorship trajectories across patients with solid tumors: An evidence-based approach. *JAMA Oncology* 4(11):1519–1526.

Eisman, A. B., A. Quanbeck, M. Bounthavong, L. Panattoni, and R. E. Glasgow. 2021. Implementation science issues in understanding, collecting, and using cost estimates: A multi-stakeholder perspective. *Implementation Science* 16(1):75.

Ell, K., B. Xie, B. Quon, D. I. Quinn, M. Dwight-Johnson, and P. J. Lee. 2008. Randomized controlled trial of collaborative care management of depression among low-income patients with cancer. *Journal of Clinical Oncology* 26(27):4488–4496.

Emamekhoo, H., C. B. Carroll, C. Stietz, J. B. Pier, M. D. Lavitschke, D. Mulkerin, M. E. Sesto, and A. J. Tevaarwerk. 2022. Supporting structured data capture for patients with cancer: An initiative of the University of Wisconsin Carbone Cancer Center survivorship program to improve capture of malignant diagnosis and cancer staging data. *JCO Clinical Cancer Informatics* 6:e2200020.

Fraher, E., and B. Brandt. 2019. Toward a system where workforce planning and interprofessional practice and education are designed around patients and populations not professions. *Journal of Interprofessional Care* 33(4):389–397.

Gabriel, P. E., A. P. Singh, and L. N. Shulman. 2023. Re-envisioning the paradigm for oncology electronic health record documentation by paying for what matters for patients, quality, and research. *JAMA Oncology* 9(3):299–300.

Gaga, M., C. A. Powell, D. E. Schraufnagel, N. Schönfeld, K. Rabe, N. S. Hill, and J. P. Sculier. 2013. An official American Thoracic Society/European Respiratory Society statement: The role of the pulmonologist in the diagnosis and management of lung cancer. *American Journal of Respiratory and Critical Care Medicine* 188(4):503–507.

Gallicchio, L., T. P. Devasia, E. Tonorezos, M. A. Mollica, and A. Mariotto. 2022. Estimation of the number of individuals living with metastatic cancer in the United States. *Journal of the National Cancer Institute* 114(11):1476–1483.

Gilbert, J. H., J. Yan, and S. J. Hoffman. 2010. A WHO report: Framework for action on interprofessional education and collaborative practice. *Journal of Allied Health* 39(Suppl 1):196–197.

Global Burden of Disease 2019 Cancer Collaboration. 2022. Cancer incidence, mortality, years of life lost, years lived with disability, and disability-adjusted life years for 29 cancer groups from 2010 to 2019: A systematic analysis for the Global Burden of Disease study 2019. *JAMA Oncology* 8(3):420–444.

Greilich, P. E., M. Kilcullen, S. Paquette, E. H. Lazzara, S. Scielzo, J. Hernandez, R. Preble, M. Michael, M. Sadighi, S. Tannenbaum, E. Phelps, K. H. Krumwiede, D. Sendelbach, R. Rege, and E. Salas. 2023. Team first framework: Identifying core teamwork competencies critical to interprofessional healthcare curricula. *Journal of Clinical and Translational Science* 7(1):e106.

Han, X., J. Zhao, Z. Zheng, J. S. de Moor, K. S. Virgo, and K. R. Yabroff. 2020. Medical financial hardship intensity and financial sacrifice associated with cancer in the United States. *Cancer Epidemiology, Biomarkers & Prevention* 29(2):308–317.

Hassett, M. J., S. Wong, R. U. Osarogiagbon, J. Bian, D. S. Dizon, H. H. Jenkins, H. Uno, C. Cronin, and D. Schrag. 2022. Implementation of patient-reported outcomes for symptom management in oncology practice through the SIMPRO research consortium: A protocol for a pragmatic Type II hybrid effectiveness-implementation multi-center cluster-randomized stepped wedge trial. *Trials* 23(1):506.

Häyrinen, K., and K. Saranto. 2005. The core data elements of electronic health record in Finland. *Studies in Health Technology and Informatics* 116:131–136.

Heitner, R., M. Rogers, and D. E. Meier. 2019. *Mapping community palliative care.* New York, NY: Center to Advance Palliative Care.

Hewitt, M., and J. H. Rowland. 2002. Mental health service use among adult cancer survivors: Analyses of the National Health Interview Survey. *Journal of Clinical Oncology* 20(23):4581–4590.

Ho, F. Y., W. F. Yeung, T. H. Ng, and C. S. Chan. 2016. The efficacy and cost-effectiveness of stepped care prevention and treatment for depressive and/or anxiety disorders: A systematic review and meta-analysis. *Scientific Reports* 6:29281.

Høeg, B. L., P. E. Bidstrup, R. V. Karlsen, A. S. Friberg, V. Albieri, S. O. Dalton, L. Saltbæk, K. K. Andersen, T. A. Horsboel, and C. Johansen. 2019. Follow-up strategies following completion of primary cancer treatment in adult cancer survivors. *Cochrane Database of Systematic Reviews* 2019(11).

HRSA (Health Resources & Services Administration). 2023a. *Health Workforce Shortage Areas.* HRSA. https://data.hrsa.gov/topics/health-workforce/shortage-areas (accessed November 28, 2023).

HSRA. 2023b. *Health Center Program: Impact and Growth.* HRSA. https://bphc.hrsa.gov/about-health-centers/health-center-program-impact-growth (accessed November 28, 2023).

HRSA. 2024. *Health workforce projections.* HRSA. https://bhw.hrsa.gov/data-research/projecting-health-workforce-supply-demand (accessed March 18, 2024).

Hudson, M. M., K. K. Ness, J. G. Gurney, D. A. Mulrooney, W. Chemaitilly, K. R. Krull, D. M. Green, G. T. Armstrong, K. A. Nottage, K. E. Jones, C. A. Sklar, D. K. Srivastava, and L. L. Robison. 2013. Clinical ascertainment of health outcomes among adults treated for childhood cancer. *JAMA* 309(22):2371–2381.

Humphreys, K., J. C. Blodgett, and L. W. Roberts. 2015. The exclusion of people with psychiatric disorders from medical research. *Journal of Psychiatric Research* 70:28–32.

IOM (Institute of Medicine). 2000. *To err is human: Building a safer health system.* Washington, DC: The National Academies Press.

IOM. 2008. *Committee on the future health care workforce for older Americans.* Washington, DC: The National Academies Press.

IOM. 2013. *Delivering high-quality cancer care: Charting a new course for a system in crisis.* Washington, DC: The National Academies Press.

IOM. 2015. *Measuring the impact of interprofessional education on collaborative practice and patient outcomes.* Washington, DC: The National Academies Press.

IOM and NRC (National Research Council). 2006. *From cancer patient to cancer survivor: Lost in transition.* Washington, DC: The National Academies Press.

IPEC (Interprofessional Education Collaborative). 2016. *Core competencies for interprofessional collaborative practice: 2016 update*. Washington, DC: IPEC.

Irwin, K. E., D. C. Henderson, H. P. Knight, and W. F. Pirl. 2014. Cancer care for individuals with schizophrenia. *Cancer* 120(3):323–334.

Irwin, K. E., E. R. Park, J. A. Shin, L. E. Fields, J. M. Jacobs, J. A. Greer, J. B. Taylor, A. G. Taghian, O. Freudenreich, D. P. Ryan, and W. F. Pirl. 2017. Predictors of disruptions in breast cancer care for individuals with schizophrenia. *Oncologist* 22(11):1374–1382.

Irwin, K. E., B. Moy, L. E. Fields, C. A. Callaway, E. R. Park, and L. Wirth. 2019. Expanding access to cancer clinical trials for patients with mental illness. *Journal of Clinical Oncology* 37(18):1524–1528.

Irwin, K. E., N. Ko, E. P. Walsh, V. Decker, I. Arrillaga-Romany, S. R. Plotkin, J. Franas, E. Gorton, and B. Moy. 2022. Developing a virtual equity hub: Adapting the tumor board model for equity in cancer care. *Oncologist* 27(7):518–524.

Islami, F., C. E. Guerra, A. Minihan, K. R. Yabroff, S. A. Fedewa, K. Sloan, T. L. Wiedt, B. Thomson, R. L. Siegel, N. Nargis, R. A. Winn, L. Lacasse, L. Makaroff, E. C. Daniels, A. V. Patel, W. G. Cance, and A. Jemal. 2022. American Cancer Society's report on the status of cancer disparities in the United States, 2021. *CA: A Cancer Journal for Clinicians* 72(2):112–143.

Johnson, M. N. 2023. Cardio-oncology and health equity: Opportunities for implementation. *JACC CardioOncology* 5(4):546–550.

Kamal, A. H., J. M. Maguire, and D. E. Meier. 2015. Evolving the palliative care workforce to provide responsive, serious illness care. *Annals of Internal Medicine* 163(8):637–638.

Kamal, A. H., T. W. LeBlanc, and D. E. Meier. 2016. Better palliative care for all: Improving the lived experience with cancer. *JAMA* 316(1):29–30.

Kamal, A. H., S. P. Wolf, J. Troy, V. Leff, C. Dahlin, J. D. Rotella, G. Handzo, P. E. Rodgers, and E. R. Myers. 2019. Policy changes key to promoting sustainability and growth of the specialty palliative care workforce. *Health Affairs* 38(6):910–918.

KFF. 2023. Uninsured rates for the nonelderly by age. https://www.kff.org/uninsured/state-indicator/nonelderly-uninsured-rate-by-age/?activeTab=map&currentTimeframe=2&selectedDistributions=adults-19-64&sortModel=%7B%22colId%22:%22Location%22,%22sort%22:%22asc%22%7D (accessed April 3, 2024).

Kroenke, K., D. Theobald, J. Wu, K. Norton, G. Morrison, J. Carpenter, and W. Tu. 2010. Effect of telecare management on pain and depression in patients with cancer: A randomized trial. *JAMA* 304(2):163–171.

Lange, M., F. Joly, J. Vardy, T. Ahles, M. Dubois, L. Tron, G. Winocur, M. B. De Ruiter, and H. Castel. 2019. Cancer-related cognitive impairment: An update on state of the art, detection, and management strategies in cancer survivors. *Annals of Oncology* 30(12):1925–1940.

MacKinnon, N. J., V. Emery, J. Waller, B. Ange, P. Ambade, M. Gunja, and E. Watson. 2023. Mapping health disparities in 11 high-income nations. *JAMA Network Open* 6(7):e2322310.

Mariotto, A. B., L. Enewold, H. Parsons, C. A. Zeruto, K. R. Yabroff, and D. K. Mayer. 2022. Workforce caring for cancer survivors in the United States: Estimates and projections of use. *Journal of the National Cancer Institute* 114(6):837–844.

Mattiazzi, S., N. Cottrell, N. Ng, and E. Beckman. 2022. The impact of interprofessional education interventions in health professional student clinical training: A systematic review. *Journal of Interprofessional Education & Practice* 30:100596.

McDonald, S. R., M. T. Heflin, H. E. Whitson, T. O. Dalton, M. E. Lidsky, P. Liu, C. M. Poer, R. Sloane, J. K. Thacker, H. K. White, M. Yanamadala, and S. A. Lagoo-Deenadayalan. 2018. Association of integrated care coordination with postsurgical outcomes in high-risk older adults: The Perioperative Optimization of Senior Health (POSH) initiative. *JAMA Surgery* 153(5):454–462.

McGuier, E. A., D. J. Kolko, M. L. Klem, J. Feldman, G. Kinkler, M. A. Diabes, L. R. Weingart, and C. B. Wolk. 2021. Team functioning and implementation of innovations in healthcare and human service settings: A systematic review protocol. *Systemic Reviews* 10(1):189.

Meyer, R. M., M. K. Gospodarowicz, J. M. Connors, R. G. Pearcey, W. A. Wells, J. N. Winter, S. J. Horning, A. R. Dar, C. Shustik, D. A. Stewart, M. Crump, M. S. Djurfeldt, B. E. Chen, and L. E. Shepherd. 2012. ABVD alone versus radiation-based therapy in limited-stage Hodgkin's lymphoma. *New England Journal of Medicine* 366(5):399–408.

Miller, K. D., L. Nogueira, T. Devasia, A. B. Mariotto, K. R. Yabroff, A. Jemal, J. Kramer, and R. L. Siegel. 2022. Cancer treatment and survivorship statistics, 2022. *CA* 72(5):409–436.

Natale-Pereira, A., K. R. Enard, L. Nevarez, and L. A. Jones. 2011. The role of patient navigators in eliminating health disparities. *Cancer* 117(15 Suppl):3543–3552.

Nekhlyudov, L., M. OMalley D, and S. V. Hudson. 2017. Integrating primary care providers in the care of cancer survivors: Gaps in evidence and future opportunities. *Lancet Oncology* 18(1):e30–e38.

NHS (National Health Service). 2013. *Innovation to implementation: Stratified pathways of care for people living with or beyond cancer. A 'how-to guide.'* https://www.england.nhs.uk/wp-content/uploads/2016/04/stratified-pathways-update.pdf (accessed March 27, 2024).

NIH (National Institutes of Health). 2023. *Nutrition as prevention for improved cancer health outcomes.* https://prevention.nih.gov/research-priorities/research-needs-and-gaps/pathways-prevention/nutrition-prevention-improved-cancer-health-outcomes (accessed November 28, 2023).

Noyd, D. H., Q. Liu, Y. Yasui, E. J. Chow, S. Bhatia, P. C. Nathan, A. P. Landstrom, E. Tonorezos, J. Casillas, A. Berkman, K. K. Ness, D. A. Mulrooney, W. M. Leisenring, C. R. Howell, J. Shoag, A. Kirchhoff, R. M. Howell, T. M. Gibson, L. L. Zullig, G. T. Armstrong, and K. C. Oeffinger. 2023. Cardiovascular risk factor disparities in adult survivors of childhood cancer compared with the general population. *JACC CardioOncology* 5(4):489–500.

NQF (National Quality Forum). 2006. *A national framework and preferred practices for palliative and hospice care quality.* Washington, DC: NQF.

Osterman, T. J., M. Terry, and R. S. Miller. 2020. Improving cancer data interoperability: The promise of the minimal common oncology data elements (MCODE) initiative. *JCO Clinical Cancer Informatics* 4:993–1001.

Patel, V. R., S. M. Q. Hussaini, A. H. Blaes, A. K. Morgans, A. B. Haynes, A. S. Adamson, and A. Gupta. 2023. Trends in the prevalence of functional limitations among U.S. cancer survivors, 1999–2018. *JAMA Oncology* 9(7):1001–1003.

Paterson, D. I., N. Wiebe, W. Y. Cheung, J. R. Mackey, E. Pituskin, A. Reiman, and M. Tonelli. 2022. Incident cardiovascular disease among adults with cancer: A population-based cohort study. *JACC CardioOncology* 4(1):85–94.

Perlmutter, E. Y., F. B. Herron, E. A. Rohan, and E. Thomas. 2022. Oncology social work practice behaviors: A national survey of AOSW members. *Journal of Psychosocial Oncology* 40(2):137–151.

Pickard, T., S. Williams, E. Tetzlaff, C. Petraitis, and H. Hylton. 2023. Team-based care in oncology: The impact of the advanced practice provider. *American Society of Clinical Oncology Educational Book* 43:e390572.

Pirl, W. F., J. A. Greer, S. W. Gregoric, T. Deshields, S. Irwin, K. Fasciano, L. Wiener, T. Courtnage, L. S. Padgett, and J. R Fann. 2020. Framework for planning the delivery of psychosocial oncology services: An American Psychosocial Oncology Society Task Force report. *Psycho-Oncology* 29(12):1982–1987.

Pradhan, K. R., Y. Chen, S. Moustoufi-Moab, K. Krull, K. C. Oeffinger, C. Sklar, G. T. Armstrong, K. K. Ness, L. Robison, Y. Yasui, and P. C. Nathan. 2019. Endocrine and metabolic disorders in survivors of childhood cancers and health-related quality of life and physical activity. *The Journal of Clinical Endocrinology & Metabolism* 104(11):5183–5194.

Prado, C. M., A. Laviano, C. Gillis, A. D. Sung, M. Gardner, S. Yalcin, S. Dixon, S. M. Newman, M. D. Bastasch, A. C. Sauer, R. Hegazi, and M. R. Chasen. 2022. Examining guidelines and new evidence in oncology nutrition: A position paper on gaps and opportunities in multimodal approaches to improve patient care. *Supportive Care in Cancer* 30(4):3073–3083.

Rawlinson, C., T. Carron, C. Cohidon, C. Arditi, Q. N. Hong, P. Pluye, I. Peytremann-Bridevaux, and I. Gilles. 2021. An overview of reviews on interprofessional collaboration in primary care: Barriers and facilitators. *International Journal of Integrated Care* 21(2):32.

Reeves, S., S. Fletcher, H. Barr, I. Birch, S. Boet, N. Davies, A. McFadyen, J. Rivera, and S. Kitto. 2016. A BEME systematic review of the effects of interprofessional education: BEME guide no. 39. *Medical Teacher* 38(7):656–668.

Rosko, A. E., C. Steer, L. C. Chien, J. Zittel, A. Artz, S. Chow, E. Plotkin, W. Dale, R. Elias, and A. E. Chapman. 2021. The Cancer and Aging Research Group (CARG) infrastructure: The clinical implementation core. *Journal of Geriatric Oncology* 12(8):1164–1165.

Roth, G. A., G. A. Mensah, C. O. Johnson, G. Addolorato, E. Ammirati, L. M. Baddour, N. C. Barengo, A. Z. Beaton, E. J. Benjamin, C. P. Benziger, A. Bonny, M. Brauer, M. Brodmann, T. J. Cahill, J. Carapetis, A. L. Catapano, S. S. Chugh, L. T. Cooper, J. Coresh, M. Criqui, N. DeCleene, K. A. Eagle, S. Emmons-Bell, V. L. Feigin, J. Fernández-Solà, G. Fowkes, E. Gakidou, S. M. Grundy, F. J. He, G. Howard, F. Hu, L. Inker, G. Karthikeyan, N. Kassebaum, W. Koroshetz, C. Lavie, D. Lloyd-Jones, H. S. Lu, A. Mirijello, A. M. Temesgen, A. Mokdad, A. E. Moran, P. Muntner, J. Narula, B. Neal, M. Ntsekhe, G. Moraes de Oliveira, C. Otto, M. Owolabi, M. Pratt, S. Rajagopalan, M. Reitsma, A. L. P. Ribeiro, N. Rigotti, A. Rodgers, C. Sable, S. Shakil, K. Sliwa-Hahnle, B. Stark, J. Sundström, P. Timpel, I. M. Tleyjeh, M. Valgimigli, T. Vos, P. K. Whelton, M. Yacoub, L. Zuhlke, C. Murray, and V. Fuster. 2020. Global burden of cardiovascular diseases and risk factors, 1990–2019: Update from the GBD 2019 study. *Journal of the American College of Cardiology* 76(25):2982–3021.

Ryan, A. M., D. G. Power, L. Daly, S. J. Cushen, Ē. Ní Bhuachalla, and C. M. Prado. 2016. Cancer-associated malnutrition, cachexia and sarcopenia: The skeleton in the hospital closet 40 years later. *Proceedings of the Nutrition Society* 75(2):199–211.

Salas, E., S. J. Weaver, D. DiazGranados, R. Lyons, and H. King. 2009. Sounding the call for team training in health care: Some insights and warnings. *Academic Medicine* 84(10 Suppl):S128-131.

Schaapveld, M., B. M. Aleman, A. M. van Eggermond, C. P. Janus, A. D. Krol, R. W. van der Maazen, J. Roesink, J. M. Raemaekers, J. P. de Boer, J. M. Zijlstra, G. W. van Imhoff, E. J. Petersen, P. M. Poortmans, M. Beijert, M. L. Lybeert, I. Mulder, O. Visser, M. W. Louwman, I. M. Krul, P. J. Lugtenburg, and F. E. van Leeuwen. 2015. Second cancer risk up to 40 years after treatment for Hodgkin's lymphoma. *New England Journal of Medicine* 373(26):2499–2511.

Shankaran, V., J. M. Unger, A. K. Darke, J. M. Suga, J. L. Wade, P. J. Kourlas, S. R. Chandana, M. A. O'Rourke, S. Satti, D. Liggett, D. L. Hershman, and S. D. Ramsey. 2022. S1417CD: A prospective multicenter cooperative group-led study of financial hardship in metastatic colorectal cancer patients. *Journal of the National Cancer Institute* 114(3):372–380.

Shay, L. A., M. Allicock, and A. Li. 2022. "Every day is just kind of weighing my options." Perspectives of young adult cancer survivors dealing with the uncertainty of the COVID-19 global pandemic. *Journal of Cancer Survivorship: Research and Practice* 16(4):760–770.

Shih, Y. T., B. Kim, and M. T. Halpern. 2021. State of physician and pharmacist oncology workforce in the United States in 2019. *JCO Oncology Practice* 17(1):e1–e10.

Shulman, L. N., L. K. Sheldon, and E. J. Benz. 2020. The future of cancer care in the United States—Overcoming workforce capacity limitations. *JAMA Oncology* 6(3):327–328.

Singh, G. K., and A. Jemal. 2017. Socioeconomic and racial/ethnic disparities in cancer mortality, incidence, and survival in the United States, 1950–2014: Over six decades of changing patterns and widening inequalities. *Journal of Environmental and Public Health* 2017:2819372.

Spaulding, E. M., F. A. Marvel, E. Jacob, A. Rahman, B. R. Hansen, L. A. Hanyok, S. S. Martin, and H. R. Han. 2021. Interprofessional education and collaboration among healthcare students and professionals: A systematic review and call for action. *Journal of Interprofessional Care* 35(4):612–621.

Stetson, P. D., N. J. McCleary, T. Osterman, K. Ramchandran, A. Tevaarwerk, T. Wong, J. M. Sugalski, W. Akerley, A. Mercurio, F. J. Zachariah, J. Yamzon, R. C. Stillman, P. E. Gabriel, T. Heinrichs, K. Kerrigan, S. B. Patel, S. M. Gilbert, and E. Weiss. 2022. Adoption of patient-generated health data in oncology: A report from the NCCN EHR Oncology Advisory Group. *Journal of the National Comprehensive Cancer Network* 20(13).

Stout, N. L., J. M. Binkley, K. H. Schmitz, K. Andrews, S. C. Hayes, K. L. Campbell, M. L. McNeely, P. W. Soballe, A. M. Berger, A. L. Cheville, C. Fabian, L. H. Gerber, S. R. Harris, K. Johansson, A. L. Pusic, R. G. Prosnitz, and R. A. Smith. 2012. A prospective surveillance model for rehabilitation for women with breast cancer. *Cancer* 118(8 Suppl):2191–2200.

Stout, N. L., A. Sleight, D. Pfeiffer, M. L. Galantino, and B. deSouza. 2019. Promoting assessment and management of function through navigation: Opportunities to bridge oncology and rehabilitation systems of care. *Supportive Care in Cancer* 27(12):4497–4505.

Stout, N. L., J. Greenfield, and S. Aulakh. 2023a. Feasibility of a clinically integrated rehabilitation therapist in a neuro-oncology clinic. *Neuro-Oncology Advances* 5(1):vdad098.

Stout, N. L., S. E. Harrington, A. Perry, M. J. Alappattu, V. Pfab, B. Stewart, and M. R. Manes. 2023b. Implementation of a cancer rehabilitation navigation program: A qualitative analysis of implementation determinants and strategies. *Journal of Cancer Survivorship*. https://doi.org/10.1007/s11764-023-01374-5.

Stout, N. L., C. Street, P. Policicchio, J. Summers, and A. Duckworth. 2023c. Implementing process improvements to enhance distress screening and management. *Supportive Care in Cancer* 31(6):351.

Strongman, H., S. Gadd, A. A. Matthews, K. E. Mansfield, S. Stanway, A. R. Lyon, I. Dos-Santos-Silva, L. Smeeth, and K. Bhaskaran. 2022. Does cardiovascular mortality overtake cancer mortality during cancer survivorship?: An English retrospective cohort study. *JACC CardioOncology* 4(1):113–123.

Sun, L., R. B. Parikh, R. A. Hubbard, J. Cashy, S. U. Takvorian, D. J. Vaughn, K. W. Robinson, V. Narayan, and B. Ky. 2021. Assessment and management of cardiovascular risk factors among U.S. veterans with prostate cancer. *JAMA Network Open* 4(2):e210070.

Takvorian, S. U., E. Balogh, S. Nass, V. L. Valentin, L. Hoffman-Hogg, R. A. Oyer, R. W. Carlson, N. J. Meropol, L. K. Sheldon, and L. N. Shulman. 2020. Developing and sustaining an effective and resilient oncology careforce: Opportunities for action. *Journal of the National Cancer Institute* 112(7):663–670.

Tannenbaum, S. I., A. M. Traylor, E. J. Thomas, and E. Salas. 2021. Managing teamwork in the face of pandemic: Evidence-based tips. *BMJ Quality & Safety* 30(1):59–63.

Taplin, S. H., S. Weaver, V. Chollette, L. B. Marks, A. Jacobs, G. Schiff, C. T. Stricker, S. S. Bruinooge, and E. Salas. 2015a. Teams and teamwork during a cancer diagnosis: Interdependency within and between teams. *Journal of Oncology Practice* 11(3):231–238.

Taplin, S. H., S. Weaver, E. Salas, V. Chollette, H. M. Edwards, S. S. Bruinooge, and M. P. Kosty. 2015b. Reviewing cancer care team effectiveness. *Journal of Oncology Practice* 11(3):239–246.

Tevaarwerk, A. J., J. R. Klemp, G. J. van Londen, B. W. Hesse, and M. E. Sesto. 2018. Moving beyond static survivorship care plans: A systems engineering approach to population health management for cancer survivors. *Cancer* 124(22):4292–4300.

Thompson, K. L., L. Elliott, V. Fuchs-Tarlovsky, R. M. Levin, A. C. Voss, and T. Piemonte. 2017. Oncology evidence-based nutrition practice guideline for adults. *Journal of the Academy of Nutrition and Dietetics* 117(2):297–310.e247.

Tollman, S. M. 1994. The Pholela health centre—The origins of community-oriented primary health care (COPC). An appreciation of the work of Sidney and Emily Kark. *South African Medical Journal* 84(10):653–658.

Trujillo, E. B., K. Claghorn, S. W. Dixon, E. B. Hill, A. Braun, E. Lipinski, M. E. Platek, M. T. Vergo, and C. Spees. 2019. Inadequate nutrition coverage in outpatient cancer centers: Results of a national survey. *Journal of Oncology* 2019:7462940.

Tsao, P. A., J. R. Fann, A. L. Nevedal, L. E. Bloor, S. L. Krein, and M. E. V. Caram. 2023. A positive distress screen . . . now what? An updated call for integrated psychosocial care. *Journal of Clinical Oncology* 41(31):4837–4841.

Tsui, J., J. A. Hirsch, F. J. Bayer, J. W. Quinn, J. Cahill, D. Siscovick, and G. S. Lovasi. 2020. Patterns in geographic access to health care facilities across neighborhoods in the United States based on data from the National Establishment Time-Series between 2000 and 2014. *JAMA Network Open* 3(5):e205105.

Tuzovic, M., S. A. Brown, E. H. Yang, B. H. West, N. S. Bassi, S. Park, A. Guha, A. K. Ghosh, S. Ganatra, S. S. Hayek, J. Moslehi, and E. Jahangir. 2020. Implementation of cardio-oncology training for cardiology fellows. *JACC CardioOncology* 2(5):795–799.

Ulrich, C. M., C. Himbert, K. Boucher, D. W. Wetter, R. Hess, J. Kim, K. Lundberg, J. A. Ligibel, C. A. Barnes, B. Rushton, R. Marcus, S. R. G. Finlayson, P. C. LaStayo, and T. K. Varghese. 2018. Precision-exercise-prescription in patients with lung cancer undergoing surgery: Rationale and design of the PEP study trial. *BMJ Open* 8(12):e024672.

Verhoeven, D. C., V. Chollette, E. H. Lazzara, M. L. Shuffler, R. U. Osarogiagbon, and S. J. Weaver. 2021. The anatomy and physiology of teaming in cancer care delivery: A conceptual framework. *Journal of the National Cancer Institute* 113(4):360–370.

Waddell, K. J., P. D. Shah, S. Adusumalli, and M. S. Patel. 2020. Using behavioral economics and technology to improve outcomes in cardio-oncology. *JACC CardioOncology* 2(1):84–96.

Walker, J., C. H. Hansen, P. Martin, S. Symeonides, C. Gourley, L. Wall, D. Weller, G. Murray, and M. Sharpe. 2014. Integrated collaborative care for major depression comorbid with a poor prognosis cancer (SMART Oncology-3): A multicentre randomised controlled trial in patients with lung cancer. *Lancet Oncology* 15(10):1168–1176.

Weaver, M. S., A. R. Rosenberg, J. Tager, C. S. Wichman, and L. Wiener. 2018. A summary of pediatric palliative care team structure and services as reported by centers caring for children with cancer. *Journal of Palliative Medicine* 21(4):452–462.

Williams, G. R., K. E. Weaver, G. J. Lesser, E. Dressler, K. M. Winkfield, H. B. Neuman, A. E. Kazak, R. Carlos, L. J. Gansauer, C. S. Kamen, J. M. Unger, S. G. Mohile, and H. D. Klepin. 2020. Capacity to provide geriatric specialty care for older adults in community oncology practices. *Oncologist* 25(12):1032–1038.

Wu, C. C., J. R. Fann, K. R. Nelson, A. R. Rosenberg, and W. F. Pirl. 2023. Collaborative care: A solution for increasing access to psychosocial care in cancer programs and practices. *Oncology Issues* 38(4):31–38.

Yabroff, K. R., J. Zhao, Z. Zheng, A. Rai, and X. Han. 2018. Medical financial hardship among cancer survivors in the United States: What do we know? What do we need to know? *Cancer Epidemiology, Biomarkers & Prevention* 27(12):1389–1397.

Yabroff, K. R., A. Mariotto, F. Tangka, J. Zhao, F. Islami, H. Sung, R. L. Sherman, S. J. Henley, A. Jemal, and E. M. Ward. 2021. Annual report to the nation on the status of cancer, part 2: Patient economic burden associated with cancer care. *Journal of the National Cancer Institute* 113(12):1670-1682.

Zhao, J., X. Han, L. Nogueira, S. A. Fedewa, A. Jemal, M. T. Halpern, and K. R. Yabroff. 2022. Health insurance status and cancer stage at diagnosis and survival in the United States. *CA: A Cancer Journal for Clinicians* 72(6):542–560.

Zheng, Z., A. Jemal, R. Tucker-Seeley, M. P. Banegas, X. Han, A. Rai, J. Zhao, and K. R. Yabroff. 2020. Worry about daily financial needs and food insecurity among cancer survivors in the United States. *Journal of the National Comprehensive Cancer Network* 18(3):315–327.

Zhu, C., T. Shi, C. Jiang, B. Liu, L. A. Baldassarre, and S. Zarich. 2023. Racial and ethnic disparities in all-cause and cardiovascular mortality among cancer patients in the U.S. *JACC CardioOncology* 5(1):55–66.

Zullig, L. L., M. Shahsahebi, B. Neely, T. Hyslop, R. A. V. Avecilla, B. M. Griffin, K. Clayton-Stiglbauer, T. Coles, L. Owen, B B. Reeve, K. Shah, R. A. Shelby, L. Sutton, M. A. Dinan, S. Y. Zafar, N. P. Shah, S. Dent, and K. C. Oeffinger. 2021. Low-touch, team-based care for co-morbidity management in cancer patients: The One Team randomized controlled trial. *BMC Family Practice* 22(1):234.

Appendix A

Statement of Task

A planning committee appointed by the National Academies of Sciences, Engineering, and Medicine will plan and host a 1.5-day public workshop that will explore opportunities to enhance collaboration and communication among clinicians in different disciplines and medical specialties who provide care for patients with cancer, from diagnosis through survivorship. The workshop will feature invited presentations and panel discussions on topics that may include

- Opportunities for collaboration and information-sharing among members of a patient's health care team across clinical specialties (e.g., oncology, primary care, cardiology, endocrinology, rehabilitation, and others) to identify best practices for care coordination and workforce utilization.
- Approaches to enhance care competencies for patients with cancer across the spectrum of non-oncology clinicians.
- Payment and care delivery models to facilitate care coordination and collaboration among oncology, primary care, and other disciplines and medical specialties
- Strategies to expand and strengthen the workforce to improve equitable access to high-quality care for patients living with and beyond cancer, particularly in rural and other underserved areas.
- Opportunities to strengthen the evidence base about the array of adverse effects of cancer and cancer treatment on patient outcomes, including the impact on multiple organ systems—as well as interventions aimed at

mitigating the adverse effects—through improved surveillance activities for patients diagnosed with cancer.

The planning committee will develop the agenda for the workshop sessions, select and invite speakers and discussants, and moderate the discussions. A proceedings of the presentations and discussions at the workshop will be prepared by a designated rapporteur in accordance with institutional guidelines.

Appendix B

Workshop Agenda

JULY 17, 2023

8:00am **Welcome and Introductory Remarks**
Planning Committee Co-Chairs:
- Larissa Nekhlyudov, Brigham and Women's Hospital/Dana-Farber Cancer Institute, Harvard Medical School
- Lawrence Shulman, University of Pennsylvania Abramson Cancer Center

8:30am **Session 1: Overview of the Cancer Care Continuum and Need for Multidisciplinary and Multispecialty Care**
Co-Moderators:
- Gwen Darien, National Patient Advocate Foundation
- Larissa Nekhlyudov, Brigham and Women's Hospital/Dana-Farber Cancer Institute, Harvard Medical School

Patient Perspectives on Multidisciplinary, Multispecialty Care
- Jacqueline Mbayo, Endometrial Cancer Action Network for African Americans
- Susan Bader
- Alia Graham, Head Up, Inc.
- Jeremy Pivor, Planetary Health Alliance, Harvard University

Overarching Challenges of Multidisciplinary and Multispecialty Expert Care for Patients Living with and Beyond Cancer
- Robert Carlson, National Comprehensive Cancer Network
- Linda Jacobs, University of Pennsylvania

The Role of Community Health Centers in Reducing Cancer Health Disparities
- Robert Winn, Virginia Commonwealth University

Workforce Considerations for Multidisciplinary and Multispecialty Patient Care
- Deborah K. Mayer, University of North Carolina at Chapel Hill

Panel Discussion

10:15am **Break**

10:30am **Session 2: Real World Examples of Providing Multidisciplinary, Multispecialty Expert Care for Patients Living with and Beyond Cancer**
Co-Moderators:
- Smita Bhatia, University of Alabama at Birmingham
- Lawrence Shulman, University of Pennsylvania Abramson Cancer Center

Cardio-Oncology
- Bonnie Ky, University of Pennsylvania

Rehabilitation Medicine
- Nicole Stout, West Virginia University

Psychosocial Health Care
- Bill Pirl, Dana-Farber Cancer Institute/Harvard Medical School

Panel Discussion with Speakers and Additional Panelists
- Primary Care: Youngjee Choi, Johns Hopkins University
- Fertility Preservation: Clarisa Gracia, University of Pennsylvania
- Endocrinology: Lillian Meacham, Emory University
- Pulmonology: Patrick Nana-Sinkam, Virginia Commonwealth University
- Nutrition: Cynthia Thomson, University of Arizona
- Cognition: Diane Von Ah, The Ohio State University

APPENDIX B

12:30pm **Break**

1:15pm **Session 3: Education and Training Opportunities**
Co-Moderators:
- Randy Jones, University of Virginia
- Larissa Nekhlyudov, Brigham and Women's Hospital/Dana-Farber Cancer Institute, Harvard Medical School

Education and Training Challenges and Opportunities for Multidisciplinary, Interprofessional Care
- Mitchell Heflin, Duke University
- Sallie Weaver, National Cancer Institute

Education and Training Strategy to Build Team-Based Care in Palliative Care
- Arif Kamal, American Cancer Society

Exemplar of an Education and Training Strategy to Build Multidisciplinary, Multispecialty Expert Care—Geriatric Oncology
- Heidi Klepin, Wake Forest University

The Virtual Tumor Board for Mental Health and Cancer Equity
- Kelly Irwin, Massachusetts General Hospital Cancer Center, Harvard Medical School

Panel Discussion with Speakers and Additional Panelist
- Anita Gupta, Johns Hopkins University

3:15pm **Break**

3:30pm **Session 4: Health System Opportunities**
Co-Moderators:
- Randall Oyer, Penn Medicine Lancaster General Health
- Susan Schneider, Duke University

Overview of Health System-Level Interventions and Financial Strategies to Facilitate Multidisciplinary, Multispecialty Expert Care for People with Cancer
- David Dougherty, University of Pennsylvania
- Amye Tevaarwerk, Mayo Clinic

Integrated Health Systems for Better Cancer Survivorship
- Farah Brasfield, Kaiser Permanente

Panel Discussion with Speakers and Additional Panelists
- Monica Gramatges, Texas Children's Hospital
- Marlyn Allicock, University of Texas, Dallas
- Catherine Alfano, Northwell Health
- Mary Reid, Roswell Park

5:30pm **Adjourn**

JULY 18, 2023

8:00am **Session 5: Overcoming Obstacles to Comprehensive Multidisciplinary, Multispecialty Expert Care: Policy, Payment, and Advocacy Opportunities**
Co-Moderators:
- Robert Carlson, National Comprehensive Cancer Network
- Robin Yabroff, American Cancer Society

Overview of the Policy and Payment Challenges to Facilitate Multidisciplinary, Multispecialty Expert Care for People Living with and Beyond Cancer
- Robin Yabroff, American Cancer Society
- Stacie Dusetzina, Vanderbilt University School of Medicine

Panel Discussion with Speakers and Additional Panelists
- Hillary Cavanagh, Center for Medicare & Medicaid Services Innovation Center
- Lawrence Shulman, University of Pennsylvania Abramson Cancer Center
- Emily Tonorezos, National Cancer Institute
- Shelley Fuld Nasso, National Coalition for Cancer Survivorship
- Jennifer Perkins, University of California, San Francisco
- Sara Rosenbaum, George Washington University

10:15am **Session 6: Concluding Discussion and Next Steps**
Co-Moderators:
- Larissa Nekhlyudov, Brigham and Women's Hospital/Dana-Farber Cancer Institute, Harvard Medical School
- Lawrence Shulman, University of Pennsylvania Abramson Cancer Center

Panelists
- Session 1: Gwen Darien and Larissa Nekhlyucov
- Session 2: Smita Bhatia and Lawrence Shulman
- Session 3: Randy Jones and Larissa Nekhlyudov
- Session 4: Randall Oyer and Susan Schneider
- Session 5: Robert Carlson and Robin Yabroff

11:20am **Concluding Remarks**
Planning Committee Co-Chairs:
- Larissa Nekhlyudov, Brigham and Women's Hospital/ Dana-Farber Cancer Institute, Harvard Medical School
- Lawrence Shulman, University of Pennsylvania Abramson Cancer Center

11:30am **Adjourn**